BMET and Clinical Engineer

Healthcare Worker

BMET and Clinical Engineer

Healthcare Worker

Alan Pakaln

BMET and Clinical Engineer

Copyright © 2021 Alan Pakaln

All rights reserved.
https://alanpakaln.com

https://jointcommissionaccreditation.org

Dedication

To BMETs and clinical engineers.

BMET and Clinical Engineer

Forward

BMET?

Clinical Engineer?

Even if you're widely read, even if you're in a tech field, you may not be familiar with these job titles. Yet, you are dependent on these job functions, let me tell you.

BMET stands for Biomedical Equipment Technician, and you may have heard of Biomedical Engineering (BME), but Clinical Engineering (CE)?

BME is generally associated with research, either university or manufacturing; though you will often find Biomedical Engineering departments in hospitals, servicing medical equipment. That's because CE is a relatively new designation.

BMETs and CEs are healthcare workers who maintain the clinical or medical technology – just about everything – that is used to treat patients in healthcare settings, nursing homes and hospitals.

BMET and Clinical Engineer

Introduction

I don't need to tell you that today, everything is a business. My career in healthcare was no exception, and that is why oversight, and understanding what is behind that process, is important: healthcare, like it or not, is a balance between risk and cost.

Hospital environments, including risk management, are multifaceted and fraught with pitfalls: anyone involved in healthcare and saying otherwise is not paying attention.

I worked in several New York City hospitals for over 30 years; I have an intuitive sense of what that environment is like. One way to judge a hospital is to look at hospitals' outcomes – infection rates, accidents, deaths, readmissions – and extrapolate from those a sense of their overall quality of care.

Another way is to look more closely at how well their assessments of risks matches their outcomes: high infection rates indicate risky behavior somewhere in the system, indicating a need to improve behavior.

Making this book

This is a story of my work life as a hospital clinical engineer. This is also a story about hospitals: how treatment services are created and managed, how technology risks are managed, and how hospitals are evaluated for the quality of services they provide.

The term biomedical engineering is relatively new, coming into existence as technology invaded medicine in the 1950s. Clinical engineering is a bit newer, and actually a subdivision of the other.

- *Bioengineering* – the study of technology and biological processes.
- *Biomedical engineering* – the development and application of technology and physiologic processes.
- *Clinical engineering* - the application (maintenance) of medical technology in clinical settings.

For me, writing about risk in relation to system and human failures (including my own) has been painful as well as somewhat of a relief. This book isn't finished, and maybe never will be. Its audience is unclear. There are topics here that may be relevant to the general reader, for example, how hospitals are accredited and what some of the problems are in how that's done. There are also topics that technically-oriented people with a penchant for abstract thinking might be drawn to, like the risk criteria, *likelihood of failure*.

Out of necessity, clinical engineering touches on issues that are both general, in its affect on people, and specific in terms of the technology in medicine: it is difficult separating the two when considering what can happen to a patient in today's fully equipped medical facility. That said I tried to keep the general and the more abstract separated as much as possible. And I've tried to be as clear as I can be.

Consider this book more as a diary than a clear rendering of how the technology of healthcare works; and certainly, it is not "medical technology for idiots."

About the Author

Alan Pakaln is a (stubborn) clinical engineer, concerned about how The Joint Commission (being the largest of four hospital accrediting organizations) oversees medical equipment maintenance in health care facilities – specifically their procedure for calculating periodic maintenance compliance. I have 30+ years experience overseeing the application of medical technology in New York City hospitals: Bellevue Hospital, St. Luke's / Mount Sinai West, and New York Presbyterian Hospital.

I have participated in Joint Commission surveys, and have previously written about this subject in a professional journal (AAMI). I have also contacted the Joint Commission regarding this issue.

I have been contacting what I consider appropriate individuals in healthcare about this issue and so far I have received very few responses. Which does and does not surprise me, given that this is not a sexy issue; it does not cry out that "lives will be saved;" nor does it lay bare some impending doom.

However, poorly maintained equipment can be involved in incidents, or contribute to confusion during procedures causing increased risk and delays in treatment.

It is also difficult confronting The Joint Commission. Most of the time, administrators and clinicians are just trying to survive in a competitive environment. The Joint Commission is a huge bureaucracy, and not always willing to listen to complaints.

On the other hand, the issue of accurate and meaningful patient care record keeping is something everyone acknowledges is critical to successful outcomes (and then there's ethics).

BMET and Clinical Engineer

Contents

Human Disconnect (**Introduction**)	1
Medical Technology: Blast Off!	9
The People's Hospital	17
Mergers - The Beginning of The End	41
Risky Business	55
Improvements	65
Trying to Make Things Better	67
It's Not a Fun Subject	77
Joint Commission Statement	83
Addendum	95
Other Books	119

BMET and Clinical Engineer

Human Disconnect

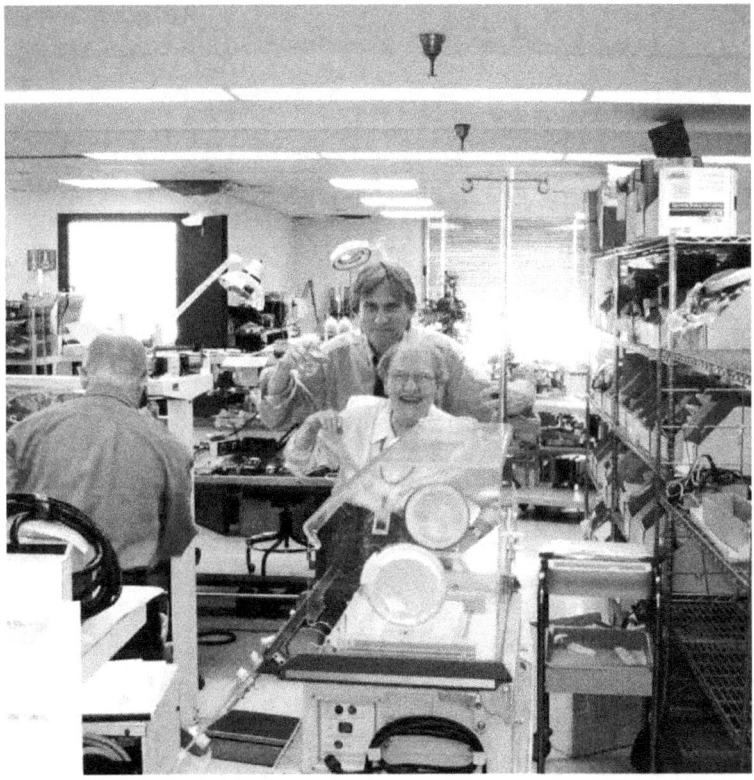

The author at work.

BMET and Clinical Engineer

Human Disconnect

Sometime in my first year of working in my first hospital, Bellevue in NYC, I thought I had a heart attack – at work. I felt a clutching in my chest, I turned pale and almost passed out. It wasn't painful, but I had never felt anything like it before.

This happened in the Biomedical Engineering department, and the staff got a wheelchair, plopped me in it and took me to the ED (What we called the ER – the Emergency Department). The director of the department asked me a few questions and then, inadvertently, introduced me to what would become my appreciation of technology's human disconnect. He pinched my thumbnail, released it, looked at me and said the following - and believe me when I say I remember his exact words – "Well, you haven't had a heart attack, but it's going to take us four hours to prove it." He then left for the next patient, and left me wondering about what had just happened.

I was a clinically-oriented technology person, familiar with medical devices and assessing the human connection to those devices, so I shouldn't be surprised by an examination. But I was. He had just pronounced me probably heart-attack-free - by using my answers to his questions plus a pinch of a fingernail. I was impressed if not entirely convinced.

An EKG and blood test followed, and the doctor's assessment was quite correct: no heart attack, just a esophageal spasm triggering vasovagal syncope: a muscle spasm affecting my nervous system and causing me to feel faint. Translation: I was experiencing a lot of stress in my new job, and not paying enough attention to it: lifestyle issues really, eating right, getting enough sleep, and watching my alcohol consumption.

Actually, I didn't fully realize the significance of this experience until years later. When the doctor pinched my thumbnail and released it, he was using a time-honored method of quickly assessing cardiac output: was my heart pumping a sufficient amount of blood? The answer, as he observed, was yes, probably. Pinching my nail pushed blood out of capillaries just under the nail and caused it to turn white or pale. When he let go of the nail, blood came rushing back and the natural pink color returned quickly, indicating a satisfactory response of my pumping system. My heart was doing what it was suppose to; I had no numbness anywhere, no pain, light-headedness was momentary: no heart attack.

This was 1979. Since then, the tools of medical technology have been increasing and increasingly taking over with one effect being the intuitive assessments of clinicians not relied on as they once were. There is a disconnect: technology is standing in between the patient and the clinician.

Is a reliance on technology in medicine a good thing? It enables greater efficiencies in assessing patients faster, it helps to standardize results for trending (a blood pressure machine will behave the same way with each test compared with different clinicians using different techniques), and machines can offer increased accuracy and improved documentation. So, yes, it can be. But a dependency on technology can leave gaps in understanding nuances – sometimes big enough to fly a jetliner through.

A September, 2019 *New York Times* article, written by William Langewiesche regarding the Boeing 737 MAX crashes, proposes that the causes of the crashes were indeed design faults in automatic systems, but also pilot error, and also a lack of pilot training. The automatic systems were effectively crippled by the absence of redundant devices, installed only as additional cost add-ons, and the lack of pilot training for the new 737 MAX was a cost-saving decision as well.

The type of auto systems Boeing relied on still required pilot intervention at critical times when systems did not perform as anticipated. Which, unfortunately, was the case in the two crashes, only the pilots had incorrect information from the on-board systems, and in any event, did not have the proper training to attempt a correction.

Boeing's main competitor, Airbus, made early design decisions that clearly distinguished it from the 737 MAX including greater emphasis on automatic flight systems, and less reliance on pilot discretion. One good reason for employing greater reliance on programmed system responses is that it can reduce crashes due to pilot error. Keep in mind that Airbus made this decision before the 737 crashes: it's just now that we can compare the two different aircraft design philosophies and make something relevant come to light.

In making their decisions, Airbus designers may have anticipated issues that can become problematic: an increase in the number of start-up airlines, increased ridership, greater ticket price competition, more planes, more pilots, and more costly training. It's possible to see how greater automation in flying an aircraft can increase efficiencies in airline costs, even as it further distances the operator from the technology.

Automated systems are not all bad, but they definitely add a new layer of interaction as well as interpretation. All susceptible to unforeseen developments.

Risk and the human disconnect

Just as an autopilot system can potentially get pilots flying in less time and save pilots from making errors, use a piece of equipment for vital signs assessments of patients instead of relying on hands-on techniques makes things move faster and can help rule out errors and inconsistencies. It all works great unless programed flight systems fail, or the patient exhibits unusual symptoms, or other unexpected conditions arise and hands-on action becomes critically necessary.

Imbedded in many services, like transportation and healthcare, are cost analyses and risk assessment. You may know what cost analysis represents, but may not realize exactly what is involved in making a risk assessment. Here's a short answer: Risk assessment is a formal practice of comparing the *likelihood* of failure - something bad happening - with the *consequence* of that failure - the ability to cause harm or some kind of loss. We might also add, how *noticeable* a failure is – perhaps something is a greater risk if you can't notice the cause of failure (Boeing's automatic system for example), and lower, if you can (good visibility while driving through an intersection). The ability to detect a potential risk early on offers an opportunity to make a correction before something bad happens.

There are many forms of risk assessment, and depending on the industry, it can be very complicated or not so much. In some cases managing risk can be troublesome or even controversial: how much control should be automatic, how much human oversight should be built in when, not if, planned functions fail?

Automatic systems are here to stay. And, at some point in time, even the best designs can fail, either due to environmental interference that goes beyond anyone's ability to control (an asteroid hit), or human failure (mental/physical illness), or just something that no one ever thought of. And when unexpected failures occur, fingers

BMET and Clinical Engineer

will point to the usual suspects: technology designs and human error. Which may not be incorrect, but can ignore the fact that, in some cases, human interaction is simply not – as a fail-safe - considered as an integral part of the design. There is a tendency to use the technological innovation and then modify how humans use the technology after it fails (Just recall the countless times cellphone technology has been modified to adjust to some discomfort).

In some ways a hospital is like an aircraft system: when staff are properly trained, the various policies and procedures work to carry out prescribed functions. In its best form these procedures accomplish this regardless of the personal views or idiosyncrasies of the staff.

When the overall design has taken into account the risks inherent in various hospital functions, and effective policies are in place to address these risks, we may have what we consider a good hospital, and can expect good outcomes. But something else is needed. What are the built-in fail-safe backups that can deal with the unexpected? Answer: personal initiative, and periodic reviews of standards and procedures.

How should hospitals be judged?

The backup for when hospital systems fail is the actions of individual staff to do the right thing - independent of the prescribed system design and the policies and procedures. Example: a housekeeper (not to pick on housekeepers!) cleans a room according to prescribed procedures, but shortly after, someone else spills something on the floor. Someone else with a different function walks by and notices the unclean room, and takes corrective action; they "interfered" to correct the problem. In any system, should the need arise, individuals must know they can act independently to avert failure: the assumption being that a system <u>will fail</u> at some future point in time.

A good hospital is an egalitarian community where most of the time everyone is working together for a common goal, the benefit of patients. Unfortunately, you can't determine the quality of that community by reading *U.S. News Best Hospitals Rankings and Ratings*, or any other report because empowering people to do the right thing requires a personal relationship.

Hospitals, nursing homes, urgent care and walk-in clinics, rehab facilities - the vast majority of these services are surveyed, and if they pass, they are accredited. All of these services utilize some form of medical technology to one degree or another.

Accreditation is something you may be aware of, and your assumption may be that the facility displaying some golden emblem has met prescribed standards of care. You may also assume that the doctors, nurses, technicians, and everyone else employed by an accredited facility, function within those standards. Those are the human being parts of medicine. What about the machines of medical technology – the monitors, EKG machines, ventilators - what is their standard of care?

You probably realize that medical technology has a major role to play in the treatment of patients. But what do you know about the safety and effectiveness of these various machines? Are they inspected? Are there safety and treatment standards. How are these standards set? And by whom? Some of the answers to these questions are probably what you would expect – yes *there are standards*. But some answers may surprise or confuse you – some standards are *designed to be passed*.

Medical technology occasionally makes headlines when new treatment modalities are introduced, like robotic surgery or a new cancer treatment. But really, medical technologies are continually evolving, pushing clinical boundaries in ways that affect every aspect of patient care.

Someone somewhere should be paying close attention to what medical technology does and how it works. The "buck stops here" at the Food and Drug Administration (FDA). The FDA is the top quality and safety authority. It is not the only participant, and in a very real sense, the FDA isn't even the most important key player.

So who is? Who assures that the machines of medicine are working the way they should?

Here, briefly, is a list of some of the sources of my sometimes painful experiences.

- The standards hospitals adhere to are evaluated by organizations approved by the Centers for Medicare & Medicaid Services (CMMS). Hospitals are periodically surveyed, and when they pass, are "accredited" and given the ability to receive CMMS reimbursements. Four organizations accredit hospitals in the U.S., and like any business, they compete on service and price - the business being accreditation. The reputations of hospitals depend somewhat on the reputations of the accreditation organizations (maybe you've seen their plaques hanging on hospital entrance walls), and the other way around: accreditation organizations benefit when their hospitals look good.

It's a self-regulated system, where accreditors and accredited both benefit when everyone looks good. And like the Federal Aviation Administration (FAA), the CMMS actually has little input to the creation or application of standards. In fact, some of these standards are *designed* so that hospitals *will* pass – more on this.

- As important as risk assessments are to the safety of patients in hospitals, there are no standards for how risks are assessed. None whatsoever. Combined with the lack of oversight by the CMMS on how standards are applied, it means hospitals are free to assess many risk any way they wish, leading to some very strange and potentially dangerous results – more on this.

Medical Technology: Blast Off!

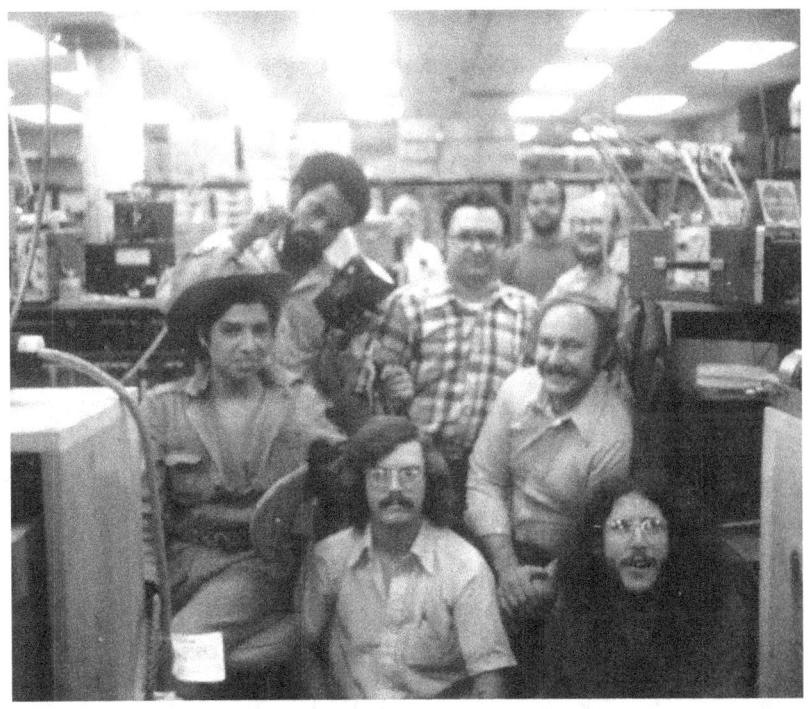

Technicians at Electronics for Medicine, c. 1978.

BMET and Clinical Engineer

Medical Technology: Blast Off!

𝓜y starting point in this field may be placed in an operating room in 1959 when I was 12 years old. A year and a half earlier I was misdiagnosed as having contracted something called ECHO virus, and was hospitalized several times: turns out I had a strangely-oriented appendix and episodes of appendicitis. How I ended up in a hospital having my appendix removed must be credited to a desperate visit to our old family doctor in the Bronx: we had traded him in for a suburban pediatrician (who almost killed me with a wrong diagnosis) when we moved out of Yonkers.

There were several key differences between the two MDs besides age and location. One was that our old family doctor performed his own white cell blood count – a measure of the degree of infection – using a microscope right there in his exam room. Another was he didn't confuse the evidence with the diagnosis. Meaning, regardless of the possibility that my disease could be ECHO related, once he probed, listened to me yelp, saw the white count, he knew the odds – "Your appendix is coming out tonight!" Picked up the old fashioned wall phone and booked me into Bronx-Lebanon Hospital.

And off we went, directly to the hospital. I can imagine my mother was concerned, but I wasn't. This was a new adventure. My take on this is that children, some children, given a lack of past experiences, allows them the opportunity of just seeing things just as they are, not as they might be or should not be. I was already taking every gadget I could find, taking it apart, and sometimes rearranging the pieces – I was technologically predisposed to see things my way, and not my mother's.

No time to waste so I'm immediately wheeled into the operating room to be prepped and opened. I remember the green walls (the trend in those days), the stainless trays, nurses, doctors, my arm being stretch out waiting for a needle. I'm looking at everything and the surgeon, while prepping is talking to me. A one point, I ask him what it takes to become a doctor. He offered a measured response intended to reassure, detailing the steps from pre-med college, to medical school, to residency, to fellowship. And then, he said, you have to pass your board exam. There was a pause, and I said, "Well I certainly hope you passed" (A bit of wisenheimer I have to this day).

BMET and Clinical Engineer

The staff broke out laughing and the surgeon says, "We've got a live one here!" And he enabled me to stay that way – alive.

This experience did not launch my career – there were many others to come - but it does speak to several issues having to do with *privilege*. Living in the New York City region gave me access to many things – available in other larger cities – things like people with a lot of experience who are willing to share it and be seen demonstrating their skills.

It's coincidence that my career path followed the development of some critical modern technologies in medicine. In 1977, I was a technician working for a company, *Electronics for Medicine (EforM)*, the first manufacturer of physiologic monitoring. Following that, in 1979, I was the assistant director of biomedical engineering at Bellevue Hospital in New York. It was here, in the early 1950s, that a prototype of the EforM monitor had been used for the first cardiac catheterization on a patient.

That story has nothing to do with me, but it was, nonetheless, an interesting path for me to have followed. The 1970s was a period when medical technology was transitioning to become a significant influence everywhere in medicine. Machine and electronic technologies were entering hospitals, and manufacturers were ramping up to meet the demand.

In 1977, my first day working at EforM was notable by the fact that I had no orientation to the job other than technicians showing me the racks of equipment that were to be assembled and tested. There were about ten of us, and it was a few weeks before I learned that one of us was the supervisor of the department. I would soon learn that there were many other outstanding features of this company of 500 employees.

EforM had its beginnings in 1950 when Martin Scheiner (or Marty as he was known) and Aaron Himmelstein developed what they called a cardiotackoscope, a device that measured and displayed waveforms of the heart's electrical activity and blood pressure. Because it could display information instantaneously on a monitor, it provided a real advantage during surgery.

Two physicians, André Cournand, and Dickinson Richards, worked together for years on various research projects involving blood pressure and heart functions. These physicians, along with Dr.

Werner Forssmann, were awarded the *Nobel Prize in Physiology or Medicine* in 1956 for their work on cardiac catheterization that used a version of the cardiotackoscope monitor and recorder. The monitors I was hired to assemble and test (IM series) were about two generations past the cardiotackoscope.

While I worked at EforM, the company moved from its original "manufacturing plant," if you can call it that - a few warehouse buildings - in North White Plains to a brand new larger facility in Pleasantville, NY. In this case, moving meant removing a lot of old equipment left from the early days of manufacturing. A lot of stuff went into dumpsters, and a lot got carted off by technicians, who like me, saw these old pieces as toys to play with.

One of the pieces of equipment I managed to pack into my station wagon was a more or less complete recorder, probably a 2nd or 3rd generation from the one used for the first cardiac catheterization.

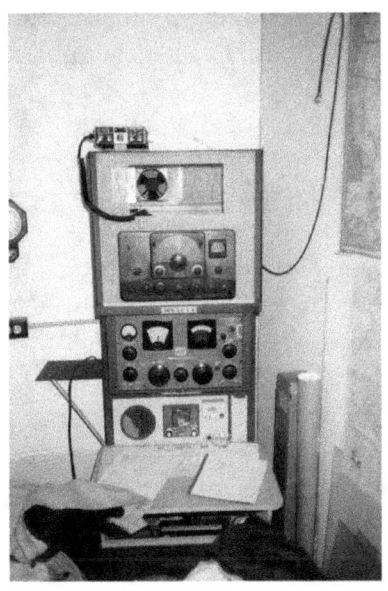

I ended up giving it to my uncle, a retired Airforce Lt. Colonel, who reconfigured it into a shortwave console, pictured here. Of course he only used the chassis, adding his components – I was impressed.

The 1979 EforM Christmas party was at the Pleasantville plant. There was food in the cafeteria, some music, and some alcohol. Behavior protocol in this company was sparse to say the least: a common expression as was explained to me went like this: "You can do anything you want, just don't insult the bosses wife." I knew who the boss was, but had no idea who his wife was; the point being, it was a very liberal work environment.

One example was this party: a technician had a bottle of mezcal, and, already in a drunken state, was looking for someone to help him finish the bottle and eat the worm (actually moth larva). He found someone and a couple of things happened. First, they shot off a dry chemical fire extinguisher in one of the test department rooms, coating the benches with powder. But then one of them through the now empty bottle into a plate glass window in the main entrance hall, shattering the glass. And, oh yes – the vice president and a few managers were in that room, and as the inebriated individual though the bottle, he shouted something like, "Damn the boss." The consequence? He was placed in a cab and sent home. He had to pay for the damaged window. That's it, and I don't remember how the extinguisher powder got cleaned up.

In the seventies and eighties, product engineering was shifting from heavy, durable, maintainable design to less of all those things, which ultimately led to more disposable products. The monitors I worked on at EforM had plug-in chips – integrated circuits – which meant, just like vacuum tubes, defective chips could be pulled and replace: quick fix, and eternally maintainable. Today, circuit boards are swapped out, cases are plastic, not steel, and new product versions can be accomplished by software updates.

EforM was developing a new updated line of equipment when it was sold to Honeywell in 1979. That was my last year, just before I left for Bellevue Hospital. Honeywell then sold this monitoring division in 1986 to the Biomedical Systems Division of PPG. In 1993-1995 PPG closed down its biomedical division. Technology manufacturing has many examples of industry leaders losing out to new businesses – like WordPerfect eventually losing to MS Word – and EforM fits that model. It died slowly, but it died.

Next steps

Medial technology has had many notable steps in development and most people have experienced some of them in personal ways. A few of these steps may have gone unnoticed even as they have impacted everyone treated in a hospital.

Explosion hazard – as in an operating room blowing up. Maybe not enough to destroy the room but enough to kill people. Ether, the primary anesthetic gas used to render a patient unconscious during surgery began to fade in use in the mid 1950s, replaced by Halothane, a nonflammable gas.

Electric shock hazard - beginning in the eighties (at least in hospitals), something called, "double insulated" devices started to be relied on. It's a design that reduces the number of electrical paths that a person can be exposed to, the effect being, a lowered risk of a patient or clinician being shocked.

Wrong medication deaths - in 2006 the FDA began a program of instituting barcodes in the process of administering medications in hospitals. That resulted in barcodes wrapped around patients' wrists and tagged on medication containers so one could be matched with the other without human interpretation and possible errors made. Fewer deaths and better treatments occur because of this procedure.

Medical error deaths - a 2016 study by Johns Hopkins suggested that 250,000 people a year may die of what's called, "medical errors." Later that estimate was reduced to 90,000, and then lowered again. The real issue is that no one really knows what the number is, and what that number stands for: there are no standards for how this data is collected or managed. More on this later.

New medical devices are developed and released to market all the time. One of the most impacting, maybe the most impacting, has been the evolution in software programming. One good example of this development is the EKG machine. In some circumstances, like in an exam room where there is a fixed laptop, the EKG functions have been "extracted" from the machine and placed in the laptop – the clinician connects the electrodes on you to the device she uses to file her report. In some applications, pulse oximeters require alarms and trending but often a finger unit can be used – buy it online for the cost of lunch.

Ultimately where all this leads is to A.I. or artificial intelligence, not only embedded in machines but managing the process of diagnosis and treatment – more than the introduction we have so far experienced. An article by Daniel Greenfield of the Harvard Graduate School of Arts and Sciences states the following:

> "The future of 'standard' medical practice might be here sooner than anticipated, where a patient could see a computer before seeing a doctor.
>
> However, while some algorithms can compete with and sometimes outperform clinicians in a variety of tasks, they have yet to be fully integrated into day-

BMET and Clinical Engineer

> to-day medical practice. Why? Because
> even though these algorithms can
> meaningfully impact medicine and bolster
> the power of medical interventions, there
> are numerous regulatory concerns that
> need addressing first."

I would never claim to know more than experts in a prestigious medical institution, but I am not persuaded that any "regulatory concerns" will hold much sway in the face of "progress" and – regardless of any Medicare for All plan - the drive for efficiency or capital investment.

It's not like the FDA turns a blind eye to medical technology; indeed they have stopped manufacturers from releasing products when safety issues arise. They can act decisively with new drugs, and device manufacturing, but when it comes to software, I question the degree of involvement: much like the FAA when it comes to oversight of aircraft auto-controls, integrity of design often falls to the more experienced manufacturers – unless or until death results.

The People's Hospital

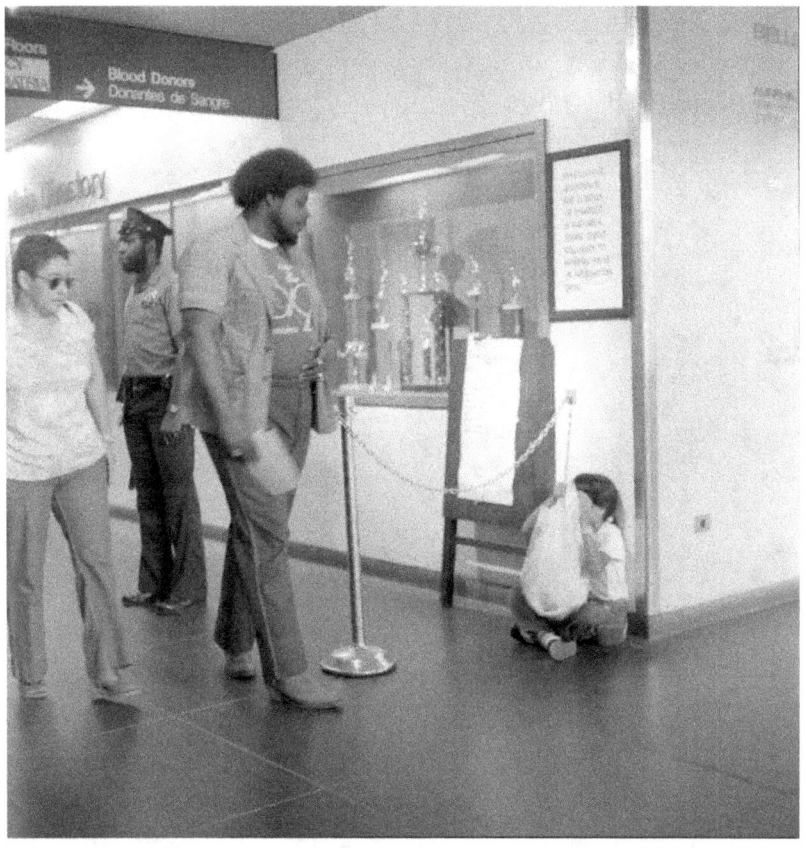

Bellevue Hospital entrance corridor, 1982.

BMET and Clinical Engineer

The People's Hospital

*B*ellevue is part of a network of New York City-owned hospitals and claims to be the oldest public hospital in America (established in 1736). It has had teaching affiliations for nursing with The City University of New York, and for physicians at NYU School of Medicine. Bellevue is one of twelve NYC Level I Trauma Centers, which basically means you can be operated on soon after you exit the ambulance - with all the services required for any contingency. Bellevue also has a prison ward, a psychiatric facility, and is next to the office of the Chief Medical Examiner. It's a big and busy place.

I wanted to work at Bellevue Hospital for two reasons. It is a big facility and I wanted a lot of different experiences: I thought that I could get it there. It is a city-owned hospital, and might not have the pretentious veneer of an upscale high-end place that only provided special treatment to a more wealthy clientele. I was right on both, and then some. I worked in Bellevue from 1979 to 1985.

I was new at hospital work and, as I consider my past, I recall a line from a play, *Hospitality Suite*: An experienced salesman is explaining the job to a young new-hire. The new guy says, "I get it, you're going to throw me into the pool and see if I can swim." The senior salesman responds, "I don't think you understand; we're going to throw you out of the plane and see if you can fly."

As the assistant director of the biomedical engineering department, I was responsible for the day-to-day operations, which included overseeing service technicians, answering service calls, and doing my share of the 24 x 7 on call response.

Anyone working in a hospital medical equipment service department is in a very unique position, one that allows a view of virtually all functions of the hospital, up close. This is true of perhaps any other person performing any other function, including doctors, nurses, and administrators.

Service personnel that test and repair medical equipment are called Biomedical Equipment Technicians or BMETs. Departments where BMETs and clinical engineers work may go by different names, typically, Biomedical Engineering, or Clinical Engineering. Clinical engineers and BMETs may be involved in a range of activities that can bring them into contact with many hospital functions, like surgical procedures, budget reviews, new technology assessments, construction of new facilities, patient injury investigations, and even the process of sterilization or of how contaminated waste is disposed.

The clinical service experience is not at all similar to academia, or working in medical equipment manufacturing, or even servicing one kind of equipment as a field service representative. It may seem obvious that, hospital environments are very different, but how different may be overlooked.

In a hospital, nurses and doctors oversee the health and wellbeing of your body, pharmacists watch over the meds you take, nutritionists watch the food, and so on, but clinical engineers and BMETs have a view of hospitals like no one else: they go everywhere, any time technology calls.

And as part of their function, they interface with administrators, clinicians, housekeepers – virtually all of the departments in a hospital.

This job is also the police force of medical technology in hospitals, always anticipating the worst, while assuring the greatest reliability of devices used on patients. I can feel overwhelmed just writing about it.

What is it like to do this job? Here are a few examples that illustrate the variety of experience.

- Managing 500 new infusion pumps in use while upgrades are made to address newly discovered problems that could - depending on some odd set of circumstances - cause a failure of the device.
- I was called by nursing to answer questions from a very cheerful patient concerning the functions of a cooling blanket. As I entered his room, he did not at first know why I was there and he asked, "Can I help you?" A visiting friend smiled and laughed. I explained how a hypo-hyperthermia machine works and we continued talking for a while about medical technology – I learned later he was receiving high levels of pain medication for cancer; the patient died that night.
- I'm having dinner at my sister's place on a Saturday evening, my pager (no cell phones yet) beeps and I call – it's a surgeon in the middle of an eye operation and the ceiling

- mounted surgical microscope jams, can't be moved into position. The tells me the electric drive motor is making noise but no movement – he does not visualize the gear and cog ceiling track so does not think about possible missing teeth in the gear. "Just manually push the microscope toward the patient, then try the motor switch." It was a guess but a good one – it worked; I went back to dinner.
- I'm speaking with a nurse in the Neuro ICU when in an empty cubicle, the electric wall outlet sparks, sparks more, then starts shooting sparks and then flames. The nurse is considering evacuating patients from the unit – not necessarily a bad choice, and something they are trained to do if necessary. But thinking there could only be a limited amount of material in the outlet that could burn, as long as the wall didn't, I asked that they wait and see (Neuro patients in intensive care can be very sensitive to movements). The flames died out. An investigation suggested the cause was the disinfectant used to wash the walls had permeated the outlet.
- A doctor calls for immediate attention in his attempt to do an EKG on a patent – the machine is broken he says, just look at the noisy trace on the print-out. I ask to see exactly how he is doing it – he screams at me, "It's the machine, just replace it." This is before stick-on electrodes, and required applying a conductive crème to an electrode plate and strapping it to the patient's arm and leg. He was using alcohol pads instead. I told him to try the crème instead, which he did and it worked. He was probably having a long day; he did apologize, and he did learn something. So did I: don't argue, explain.
- I'm in the biomedical engineering department when the secretary says I should talk to a caller – they want a fire extinguisher, she says. Could I bring one right away to the prison ward, they have a fire (Bellevue not only has a psych unit but also a treatment center for those in lock-up). Someone there called the department that made most sense to them – engineering – but did not call the fire department. I responded appropriately, telling our secretary to call the fire department, and grabbed an ABC extinguisher and off I ran.

Entering the ward was a bit surrealistic: smoke was in the air, and prisoners were pressed against the bars staring out, as I would have done under the circumstances. The fire was in a wall set off by welding that went wrong; someone grabbed the extinguisher and extinguished the fire.

- I get a call from a BMET investigating a call in the CCU. The technician tells me a nurse is frightened when testing a defibrillator – she holds the paddles apart, presses the test button, and sees a lightening bold flash across the two paddles. The technicians tells me, she is correct – there is a flash of an arc. I am not at all convinced, and proceed to the CCU, where I find the nurse and technician staring intently at the defibrillator. I repeat the test, and see a flash, but it is emanating from inside the paddles – the nurse and technician just connected the two flashes with a bolt of lightening that went between the two paddles: case solved.

There are many more examples. And though any service person in a large institution has stories to tell, you'll likely never see many from the view a hospital clinical technician has.

I selected Bellevue because, in my idealistic view, it was a hospital "for the people" so to speak. In other words, they weren't just in it for the money: true, at the time. In retrospect, I think I would have been happier working in a medium sized community hospital. It just would have seemed less overwhelming to me, less stressful, but then again.

One year, an associate director of nursing asked me to contribute photographs for the 1981-1982 Bellevue School of Nursing Bulletin. Some of the photographs shown here are from that project; others I took on my own.

The People's Hospital

Joint Commission survey for accreditation.

Now this is 1980 or so, so you must realize that things have changed since then, in all the ways they can: everyone involved have become much more sophisticated and professional in their outlook – it's a different world for sure. That said.

Survey time and the visiting surveyor (combined state and accreditation survey) is in our department – Biomedical Engineering – he will be looking at our books, but before he does that, he asks the department director to accompany him to the hospital director's office for a chat.

An hour late he returns with the Biomed Director. The surveyor smells of liquor. I later learn that a strategy of the hospital Director was to offer drinks to critical participants prior to their inspections. In our case, this strategy worked like a charm: my director and I watched as the surveyor flipped through our policy manual, pages at a time, while talking about his experiences in Paris after the war.

Very instructional?

Nothing can go wrong

Sometime during this period, Bellevue moved its phone system into the digital age: computerized. Announced of course with great fan-fare: new features, cost savings, faster response times, and so on. My director raised a concern: "What happens when the computerized system goes down?"

One should appreciate what computers were like at this time. The cardiac catheterization lab was computerized, but to describe its functionality would be similar to the Star Trek movie where Scotty is back on Earth in the Twentieth Century (*Star Trek IV: The Voyage Home*), approaches a computer consul and speaks a verbal command: "Computer...hello computer..."

The Cath lab computer had to be manually booted. "Booting up" a computer means that an initial set of software instructions are loaded into memory, volatile chip memory. Today, booting instructions are themselves stored in a chip, but back then, the Cath lab booting instructions had to be manually entered to get things going. That meant entering a particular set of numbers that were set by rotating dials.

The new phone system was a step beyond that old Cath lab

computer, and so, the administration had great expectations regarding it operation - one being, they were certain of its infallibility. "What happens when the system fails?" Answer: it won't; it can't, the system has redundancy, it is reliable.

And you know what happened, don't you? Months after its inauguration, the system went down for hours, forcing everyone to scramble setting up a paper message network to communicate between essential units. Weeks later, individual hard-wired land-lines were installed in critical units – for emergency use.

Lesson learned?

The People's Hospital

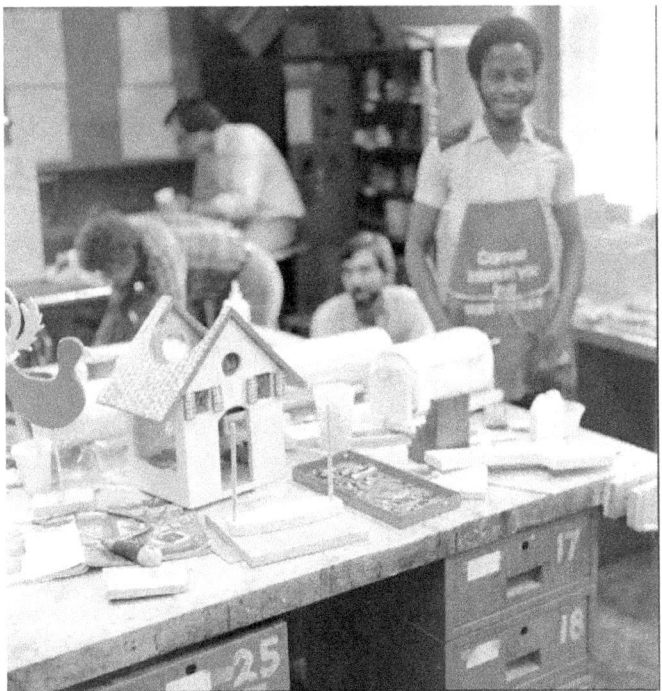

Wood workshop in Psychiatry.

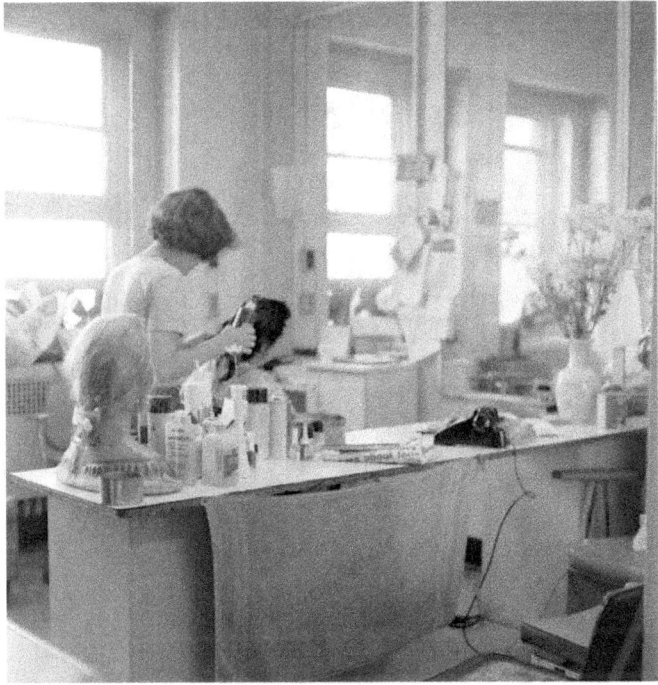

Hair salon school in Psychiatry

BMET and Clinical Engineer

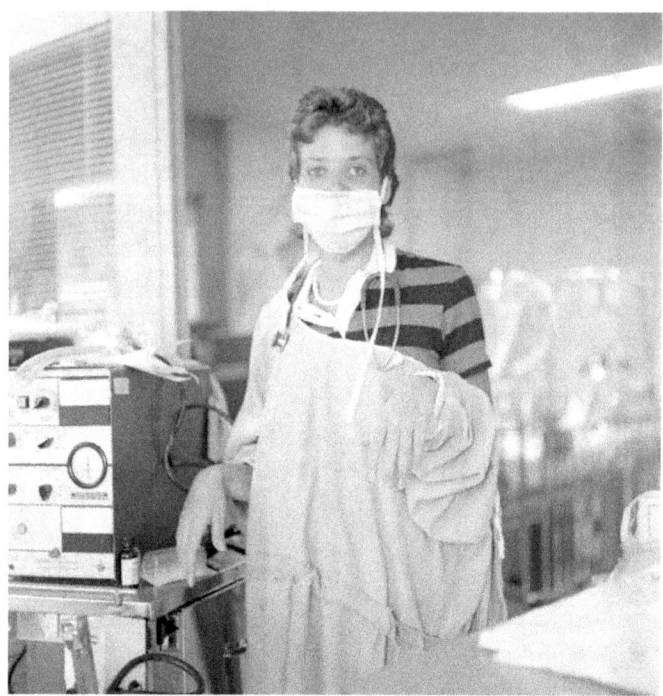

Neonatal ICU nurse.

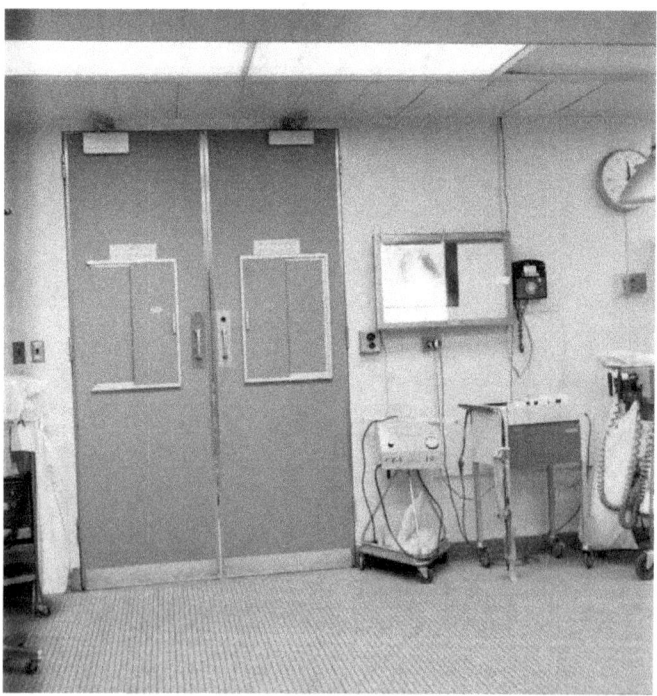

Trauma OR in ER

An Incident

A retrospective – what you do as you get older – look-back to a major event in the first 6 months of my new career: I take you back to 1979 and my introduction to patient safety and reporting.

October, 1979. The Biomedical Engineering department received a call that an external pacemaker was not functioning in the CCU procedure room. I arrived with a Medtronic pacemaker tester and found cardiologists attempting to stabilize a 57 year old male patient who had begun experiencing repeated and prolonged ectopic beats (otherwise healthy, in for pacemaker implant).

Clinicians tried 3 pacemakers and 3 pacing electrodes, with no capture spike on EKG strip. All external pacemakers tested OK. The patient continued to deteriorate – they were now defibrillating. I decided to take one of the sets of electrodes and pacemakers back to our lab for further examination.

While riding in the elevator I tried connecting the electrode to the lead wire connecting block, and found that the electrode did not appear to be fully inserted (a section of electrode contact area was exposed). In the lab, I confirmed this using an ohm meter, and quickly returned to the CCU treatment room only to find that the patient had expired (Had I noticed this during the resuscitation attempt, the outcome may have been different).

Later examination of the lead wire connection block on several new units showed a molding irregularity on the lead wire end of the block. All of the units inspected had a plastic molding of a lesser diameter on that side.

BMET and Clinical Engineer

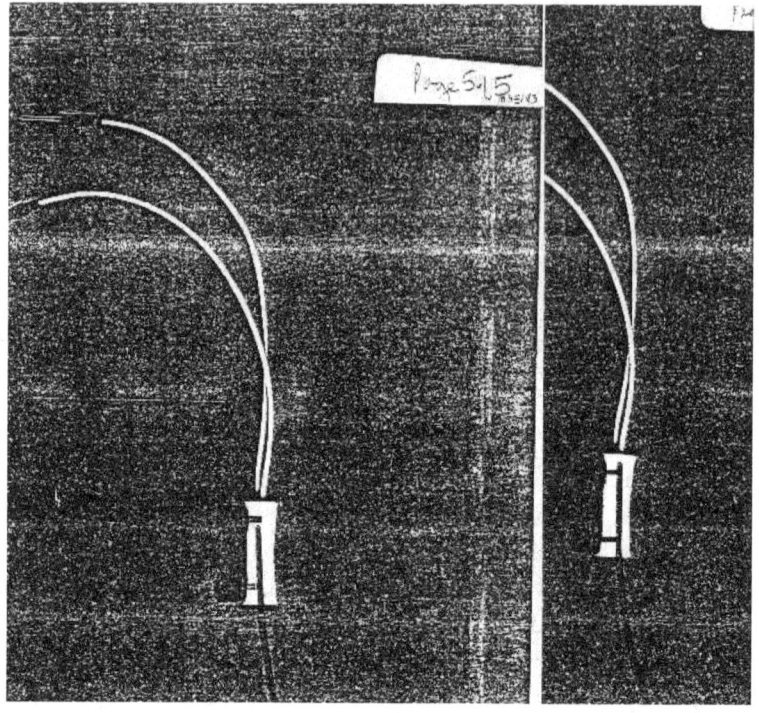

INSERTION INSTRUCTIONS
ELECTRICAL CONNECTION

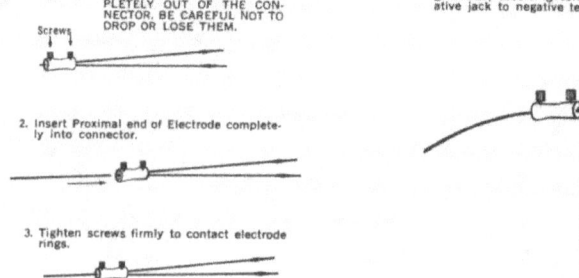

1. Loosen connector screws.
   CAUTION: SCREWS WILL COME COMPLETELY OUT OF THE CONNECTOR. BE CAREFUL NOT TO DROP OR LOSE THEM.

2. Insert Proximal end of Electrode completely into connector.

3. Tighten screws firmly to contact electrode rings.

4. Attach proximal connector jacks to pulse generator, observing correct polarity (Negative jack to negative terminal).

Out of the sterile wrap, if both screws were backed off the same number of turns, because plastic base diameter was smaller on one end, the tip of one screw would not back out as much as the other. In other words, because the end screw was effectively seated lower in the block, the same number of turns would result in the electrode passing under the first screw, but would butt up against the 2nd, thus not making positive contact with that connector.

We submitted this x-ray of the actual product plus a drawing along with our report.

The patient died – with the director of cardiology and many residents attending in the procedure room. Their assumption at the time was that the electrode pacing did not capture because it had been placed in massively infarcted tissue – "electromechanical dissociation."

Wrong. I informed the cardiologists what had happened, but the hospital director initially refused to report the incident to the FDA. Shown here is the initial notice to the hospital director.

BMET and Clinical Engineer

NEW YORK UNIVERSITY MEDICAL CENTER
School of Medicine
550 FIRST AVENUE, NEW YORK, N.Y. 10016
AREA 212 679-3200
CABLE ADDRESS NYUMEDIC

Department of Medicine

November 2, 1979

TO: Ms. Madeline Bohman

FROM: Dr. Jacob I. Hirsch

VIA: Mr. Gilbert Brooks

SUBJ: Hazardous problem associated with U.S.C.I. pacing catheter and its adapter, Cat. No. 008155

On Monday, October 29, 1979 a patient in the 17 South CCU, ▬▬▬▬▬▬, Unit # 73-59-02 expired after a cardiac arrest from which he could not be resuscitated. The medical and nursing staff were unable to pace him despite resorting to three different sets of pacing catheters and adapters of the kind noted above. It was only when one of the biomedical engineers, Mr. Alan Pakaln, was carrying one of the units down to the biomedical engineering laboratory to carry out continuity and other tests at the end of the attempts to resuscitate the patient, that he happened to notice that the catheter was not fully inserted into the adapter which allows it to be connected to the external pacemaker. It was this failure that was responsible for the pacing impulse not reaching the myocardium. All other components and factors involved were structurally and functionally intact.

The catheters included in these sets are well designed and constructed. They are 6-F, sterile, catheters of the NBIH type, with bipolar electrodes. The adapter is a white, opaque device with an opening for insertion of the proximal catheter tip and two set screws that must first be loosened to allow the catheter to be inserted, and which must then be tightened down to make contact with the two sleeve contacts on the catheter. Inspection revealed that the screw nearer the mouth of the opening is shorter that the more deeply situated screw. If the more distal screw is not loosened _more_ than the proximal screw, the tip of the catheter will abut against the distal screw, preventing full insertion, and when the screws are then tightened, they will not come down against both contacts and an open circuit will result. The opaque material of the adapter prevents visualization of this condition, yet the operator may be unaware of the problem since it feels as if the catheter is fully inserted. Dr. Paul Deutsch of our Cardiology staff, who is Director of Cardiology at St. Clare's Hospital informed me that he had similar problems with these adapters. I understand that these U.S.C.I. units are available in Bellevue Hospital only in the Cardiac Catheterization Laboratory, and I assume that it was this source that provided these units to the CCU. The rest of the hospital uses Cordis pacing catheter sets.

The problem has been discussed with Mr. Michael Mirsky, Mr. Alan Pakaln and Ms. Alice McGloin of Biomedical Engineering and with Dr. Fred Feit of the catheterization laboratory. I also called U.S.C.I. and informed a Mr. Richard Hogan of the problem. We are obliged to report this product failure to the Medical Device and Laboratory Product Problem Reporting

Program (PRP). This is a joint program involving the FDA, USP and the American College of Physicians. I have enclosed copies of the literature and reporting form. There is also a phone number to call to report such problems: (800) 638-6725.

I have refrained from reporting this until you and Mr. Brooks have been informed. Please advise me about we should now proceed. Meanwhile, I strongly urge that these adapters _not_ be used in Bellevue Hospital. As I mentioned earlier, the catheter itself is an entirely satisfactory item. I should also mention that this item did not come before the Product Evaluation Committee. Without attempting to invoke hindsight wisdom, I am certain that Mr. Mirsky and I would both have objected to its acceptance for use in Bellevue Hospital.

The People's Hospital

I filed a report to the FDA from my home.

```
PROBLEM REPORTING PROGRAM                              DATE
                                                       14
1. TRADE NAME AND TYPE OF PRODUCT (Attach labeling, if available)
   Bipolar Pacing Electrode                    November 18, 1979
2. PRODUCT IDENTIFICATION
   LOT NO.              SERIAL NO.             PRODUCT NO.
   07F94367             314620                 008155
3. NAME AND ADDRESS OF MANUFACTURER
   USCI Cardiology and Radiology Products
   Box 566
   Billerica, Ma 01821
4. EXPIRATION DATE (If applicable)

5. YOUR NAME
   Alan Pakaln (in confidence) 541 Warburton Ave. Hastings, NY 10706
6. YOUR FACILITY'S NAME, ADDRESS, AND ZIP CODE
   Bellevue Hospital Center
   NYC, NY  10016

   AREA CODE AND PHONE NUMBER OF YOUR FACILITY
   Home phone # (914) 478-4429
7. PROBLEMS NOTED OR SUSPECTED
```

The problems, I believe, are two-fold. First, a manufacturing defect. Of the two "securing" screws, the second to come in contact with the electrode must be backed off more than the first in order to allow for complete passage of the electrode as it is being inserted into the connector. We have found that with all of this type of electrode at our hospital, if both screws are loosened equally, the electrode will buttress up against the second screw and when tightened down, will in most casxes, not make electrical contact (Contact with the screw being essential for electrical continuity). The apparent cause is the difference in diameter of the moulded connector from one end to the other. Because the plastic is thinner under the second screw, it allows that screw to be posxitioned further down on the threaded conductive hole. When both screws are backed off equally, the second screw is seated lower and will block passage of the electrode. On the electrodes we have checked, the second screw must be backed off more than twice the number of turns as the first. Again, the net result is only partial or no electrical contact when installing this electrode in a usual manner.

The second problem I refered to is that of engineering design. As the enclosed Insertion Instructions state:"CAUTION: SCREWS WILL COME COMPLETELY OUT OF THE CONNECTOR. BE CAREFUL NOT TO DROP OR LOSE THEM." Furthermore, I believe that even without a manufacturing defect, the design of this device can still allow the same type of incomplete

```
1/ Additional forms and postage paid envelopes will be mailed to you at the above address when report is received.
                    United States Pharmacopeia
                    12601 Twinbrook Parkway
   RETURN TO        Rockville, Maryland  20852
                    Attention: Dr. Joseph G. Valentino
```

interconnection to be made (especially in a crisis situation) and therefore suggest that this type of 2 piece electrode be removed from the market altogether.

You will notice that I have stated (in confidence) on the face of the form. The hospital director and staff have been notified and the product was removed weeks ago but as yet I have received no word as to there intent to report this any further and I am not sure if, as you put it, my "participation is consistent with any policies that may exist in your organization". However, I am most interested in the outcome of any such action and would gladly participate further if necessary.

BMET and Clinical Engineer

	Form Approved; OMB No. 57-R0059
MEDICAL DEVICE AND LABORATORY PRODUCT PROBLEM REPORTING PROGRAM 14	ACCESS
	DATE

1 TRADE NAME AND TYPE OF PRODUCT (Attach labeling, if available)

Bipolar Pacing Electrode

2 PRODUCT IDENTIFICATION
LOT NO: 07F94367　　SERIAL NO: 314620　　PRODUCT NO: 008155

3 NAME AND ADDRESS OF MANUFACTURER
USCI Cardiology and Radiology Products
Box 566
Billerica, Ma 01820

4 EXPIRATION DATE (If applicable)

5 YOUR NAME
Alan Pakaln, Assistant Director, Biomedical Engineering

6 YOUR FACILITY'S NAME, ADDRESS AND ZIP CODE
Bio Medical Engineering Dept.
Bellevue Hospital Center
1st Ave, 27 St
NY, NY 10016

AREA CODE AND PHONE NUMBER OF YOUR FACILITY
(212) 561-6532

7 PROBLEMS NOTED OR SUSPECTED
The manufacturer has requested additional information regarding the measuring procedures used in the origonal evaluation. In answer to their questions I would like to review a functional approach and then outline my procedures.
First, the problem. When the device is removed from the sterile wrap, the screws must be backed off to permit insertion of the electrode. If the screw closest to the wired end (2nd screw) is backed off less than the one at the insertion end (1st screw) the connector may allow the electrode to pass only beneath the 1st screw but be stopped by the 2nd screw. Then, when the screws are tightened down, definite electrical contact is only possible at the first screw and may be missed there as well. To the observer, however, the electrode is attached and the screws are tight. Furthermore, since the connector is opaque, no direct visual check can be made. The only visual difference between a completely mated connection and an incomplete one is a small section of the electrode contact point petruding from the connector. For a device of this type to have functional variables at key points necessary for positive interaction with little chance for visual confirmation is, I believe, design fault.
Now there is an additional problem which I have previously refered to

RETURN TO
United States Pharmacopeia
12601 Twinbrook Parkway
Rockville, Maryland 20852
Attention: Dr. Joseph G. Valentino

OR

CALL TOLL FREE ANYTIME
800-638-6725*
IN THE CONTINENTAL UNITED STATES
*In Maryland, call collect (301)881-0256 between 9:00 AM and 4:30 PM

FORM FD 2519f (5/77)

as manufacturing defect, and this is where the measurement comes in. But, again in practical terms and refering to my new drawing:
On the electrodes that we have, we can easily see that the thickness of the plastic in the connector screw hole(c) is different at each end. And we know, from disassembling one connector, that the outside diameter of the immersed metal contacts is identical. Now this means that the 2nd screw, when fully screwed in, has made a greater penetration of the electrode path than the first, due entirely to the lesser diameter of the plastic wall at c and will take more turning than the first screw to allow for passage of the electrode. And this does happen in a practical test.
Ok, now the measurements:
All were performed using a Dial Caliper #505-626 with depth gauge, made by Mitutoyo. The depth gauge was inserted to the top of the immersed metal contact. At the 2nd screw, 40 thousandths was recorded. At the 1st, 70 thousandths of an inch.

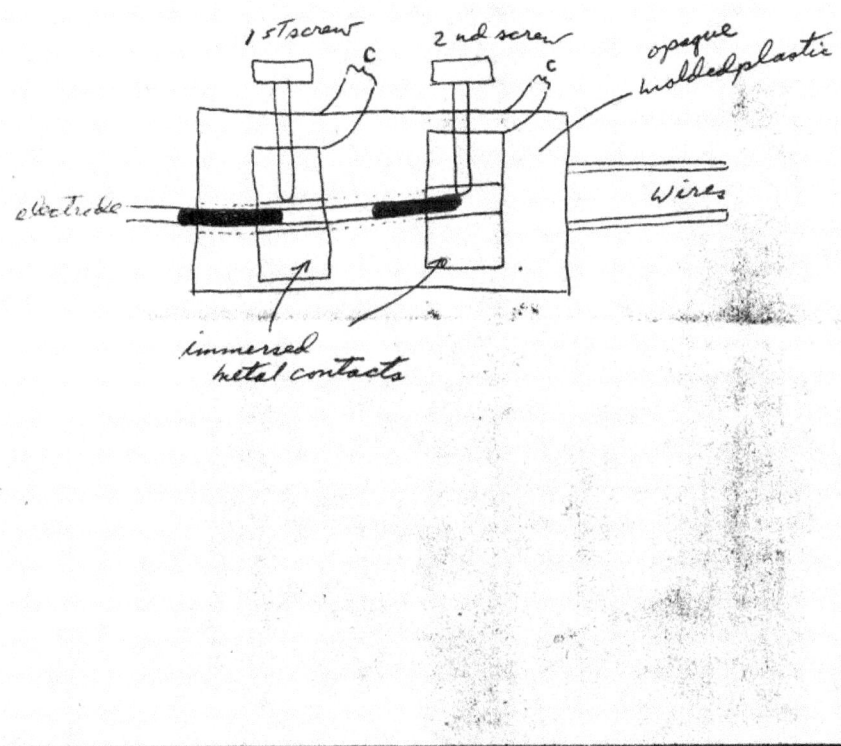

BMET and Clinical Engineer

Eventually the official hospital report was released. After some back and forth, this was the conclusion.

The People's Hospital

U. S. PHARMACOPEIAL CONVENTION, INC.
12601 TWINBROOK PARKWAY, ROCKVILLE, MD. 20852
(301) 881-0666

BOARD OF TRUSTEES

PRESIDENT
Frederick E. Shideman, M.D., Ph.D.

VICE-PRESIDENT
Harry C. Shirkey, M.D.

PAST-PRESIDENT
John A. Owen, Jr., M.D.

TREASURER
Paul F. Parker, D.Sc.

REPRESENTING MEDICINE
Arthur H. Hayes, Jr., M.D.
Leo E. Hollister, M.D.

REPRESENTING PHARMACY
William H. Barr, Pharm.D., Ph.D.
William J. Kinnard, Jr., Ph.D.
  Chairman of the Board

AT LARGE
John T. Fay, Jr., Ph.D.
Irwin Lerner

EXECUTIVE DIRECTOR
AND SECRETARY
William M. Heller, Ph.D.

April 20, 1981

Alan Pakaln
Assistant Director
Biomedical Engineering
Bellevue Hospital Center
First Avenue and 27th Street
New York, NY 10016

Dear Mr. Pakaln:

    We have received your letter requesting follow-up information on your November, 1979 report on the Bipolar Pacing Electrode.

    It is our understanding from the Food and Drug Administration that an FDA field inspection at USCI took place on March 13, 1980. The firm stated they had received no similar reports of poor electrical contact and that testing of the reported unit had found it to be working and within specifications. The FDA indicated that the firm believed the problem was due to technique error and that the labeling would be revised to detail proper technique.

    If this does not fully address your concern, please do not hesitate to bring it to our attention.

    Thank you for participating in PRP. If we may be of further assistance to you, please let us know.

Sincerely,

Deborah L. Penrod, R.Ph.
Project Coordinator,
Practitioner Reporting System

DLP:efw

Report #M-35183

The United States Pharmacopeial Convention comprises representatives from colleges and national and state organizations of medicine and pharmacy. It publishes the U.S. Pharmacopeia and the National Formulary, the legally recognized compendia of standards for drugs.

Here is the end of this story:

Several months later, a new USCI salesman shows up. When asked about this product, he explains that, yes, the item is still shown in their catalog, but, "I can assure you that none leave our loading dock." He then parroted the company line about there being no problem – we handed him a new package for him to demonstrate that there is no problem. I sometimes wonder how this affected him: he did it wrong; his patient would not have been paced.

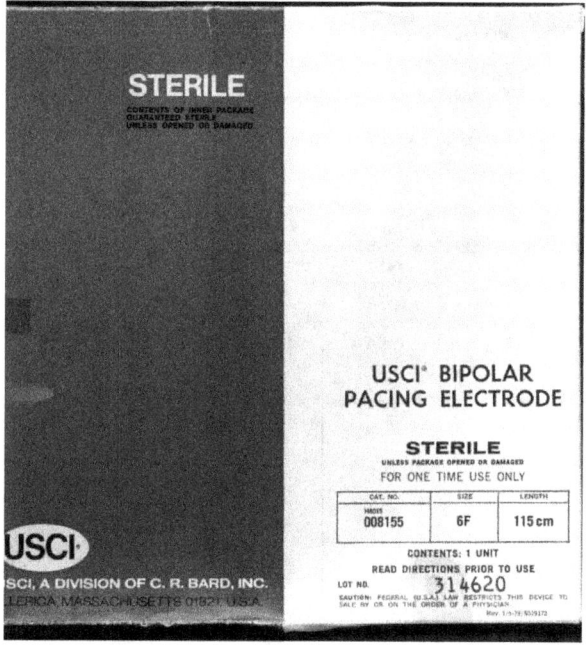

Panic Attacks

About six months after this incident - but not directly related to it - I started having severe panic attacks. The cause was a combination of factors, like the stresses of this job, and some of my own making - lifestyle. They faded out over the next 4 years.

The panic attacks actually began with physical symptoms. I was in the biomedical engineering lab working on a piece of equipment when out of the blue, I experienced a clutching sensation in my chest and then turned pale and felt faint. Oh boy – a heart attack I thought.

Symptom-wise, this was not necessarily what one might expect when having a heart attack, and though I knew that, it was sudden, strange, and frightening enough that I didn't think much. Neither did my coworkers, nor the department director. A wheelchair was brought and away I went to the emergency room.

It's kind of embarrassing being treated in the place you work. The ER determined I did not have a heart attack. But this was only the beginning of an experience that would, among other things, teach me the value of a healthy lifestyle and managing stress. The problem with my lifestyle was this: not enough sleep, poor quality sleep, drinking too much alcohol to manage stress, too much focusing on career, not enough on socializing. I was lonely and didn't really know it.

Here's the sequence of events. After my ER experience, I went back to work after taking a few days off. Lunchtime. I went out of the building with a coworker and was standing on line in a bank filling in some details of my experience of the past few days. At some point in my description, I suddenly had, what I later learned, was a severe panic attack. The intensity literally caused my knees to buckle.

In that instant, everything changed – from my perceptions of my surroundings, to how I saw my life: lights were brighter, sounds were louder, and I was surrounded by fear.

Suddenly – I could not even go back into the building after the first attack. I called a nurse friend and asked her to inform my director I was going home. I took 2 weeks off from work. These two weeks were spent going to doctors, and a psychiatrist in a crisis clinic where ironically, the doctor who was volunteering there also worked at Bellevue!

Initially, I had no idea what was happening to me. I remember asking doctors, "Am I experiencing burn-out?" Total naivety: panic attacks to the uninitiated are a unique experience difficult to explain. The psychiatrist at the clinic listened and took out his big book of disorders, thumbed through it and pointed to a paragraph: "Yup, that's it!" I had found a name for what was happening to me, and that did help. It is somewhat reassuring to know that I am not the only visitor from another "planet." Even if no other pharmaceutical help could be offered.

The panic attack has a unique quality from plain fear or what I think most people mean by anxiety. Panic is a very fast and out of control elevation of fear – and it peaks – fear is all there is for one moment. And it is exhausting to experience. Literally exhausting, leaving less energy to do anything, like think about what has just happened. One of the early attacks might take hours to recover from, before the next. Initially, I could even be wakened from sleep by a panic attack. There was no escape.

One valuable piece of advice was offered by a nurse, over the phone no less. She said something very simple yet very effective: "Stay with people." That was it. But she knew what she was talking about, and if I could I would thank her.

Doctors prescribed Valium, which I would hold in my hand as I went back out into the world, as a security blanket. Not only was this drug not very effective but as I learned, it could actually precipitate a panic attack on its own because it made me feel less in control, not more. A few other "strange" effects of attacks were: just telling a white lie could trigger an attack (increased stress level), and although alcohol consumption looked very attractive – it could elevate stress – the overall effect was to push back any stress an that could increase the likelihood of an attack.

So that was that: no drinking? Nope: it takes time for stupidity to fade. And learning can take repetition – keep making the same mistakes until you either learn to admit the truth, or become bored with the repetition. Truth is, I was struggling to keep my head above the surface of my job responsibilities, while adjusting my lifestyle habits like reestablishing social contacts, changing my diet, forcing myself to get to be earlier even though I needed to decompress after work. My brain had learned a new way of elevating stress, like a fuse blowing, or pressure valve letting go. I was not – yet – letting myself release stress a little at a time; it would build up to a point when it would pop – suddenly – and leave me wilted.

Today, there are drugs, and therapy, and much more knowledge of these kinds of experiences. In the early 1980s, the awareness of what panic attacks were and how to deal with them was in its infancy. Today there is more awareness of stress in work environments.

All the lessons I needed to learn are valid for anyone managing a stressful set of responsibilities. You know what these jobs are – fire fighting, policing, dentistry, bus drivers, and many many more. So I don't mean to single out hospital work as having greater stress on workers than other jobs, but hospital is what I know. What I personally found having the greatest positive impact on making my job less stressful – besides taking better care of myself – was the sense of community support within the institution.

I would argue that the single most important aspect contributing to a healthy hospital, and therefore its patients, and workers, is the connection everyone can feel towards one and other. Want to enable a workforce? Encourage genuine communication – the key word being *genuine*.

Mergers, the Beginning of the End

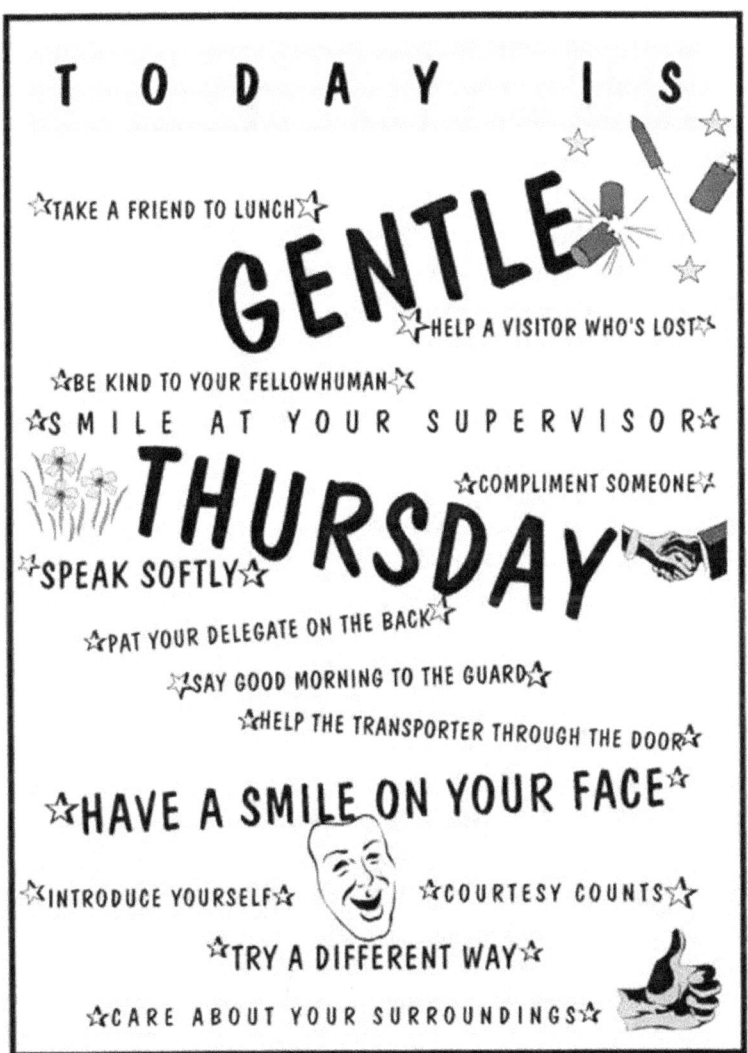

Mergers, the Beginning of the End

*I*n 1984 I walked into St. Luke's Hospital in New York City as a new hire and was yelled at as I crossed a picket line to get into the building. United Healthcare Workers, 1199, had struck the hospital, and my first two weeks were spent, days, in the biomedical engineering department, and nights as a bus-boy serving private patients in the upscale wing – seven days a week.

```
October, 1979, New York Times. "New York
City's largest private, voluntary
hospital was created yesterday with the
merger of St. Luke's and Roosevelt on the
West Side. The merged hospital, called
St. Luke's Roosevelt Hospital Center,
became the first in the city to agree to
reduce its annual operating budget by 4
percent over the next three years. It
will do so under an experimental
reimbursement program sponsored by New
York State health officials."
```

My department consisted of two CE technicians who barely tolerated each other, one of them wanted the job I was just hired into – assistant director – the other threatened to "throw you (me) out the window" when I announced that piles of accumulated equipment would be no longer be the acceptable method of resolving defects.

And St. Luke's had just merged with Roosevelt Hospital, three miles away which is where my director's office was. I was alone, over my head and scared. I worked there for 18 years, eventually overseeing the staff at both sites. It was one of the most fascinating and rewarding experiences of my life.

St. Luke's is one of those "border" hospitals, a nonprofit institution situated between lower and higher income neighborhoods on the upper west side of Manhattan, just across the street from Columbia University. It's an old institution, created in 1854 on 54th Street and 5th Ave. It moved to its current location in 1896 to 116 Street and Amsterdam Ave. in an area called Morningside Heights.

"Mergers, the beginning of the end." The end of what? Some readers may be old enough to recall what healthcare was like before hospitals became large competing networks. When patients had a "home" in a *community hospital*. Before HMO employees had a 401K, but had a pension.

Of course I can only account for what my life was like, at that time, and at that place, but I'm sure there were similar experiences in hospitals throughout this country – not withstanding being able to laugh at familiar scenes depicted in the early 2000s TV series, *Scrubs*.

BMETs had the mental space and enough free time to be able to establish lasting personal relationships. And as for my position as an administrator, that extended to other administrators; we formed a team, based as much on personal relationships as anything else.

In most large institutions there probably are big qualitative differences between the social life towards the bottom, and that life nearer the top. Not to be too crude about this, but I'm talking about the differences between working class ability to socialize and personally connect, and the owner or management ways of personally connecting.

Which group will appear more at ease chatting it up over beers at a local pub, those stocking the shelves at a distribution center, or those seated at that company's board meeting?

The Beginning

Change on The Wings of Dinosaurs.

The call went out: All managers of all departments are required to attend lunch-time meetings, each day for one week – lunch supplied. The occasion was the oncoming of HMOs (Health Maintenance Organization). Our hospital president saw the potential for this wave (1980s) to cross the country from its early beginnings in California. Which it did. And she knew that one way or another, everyone working in a hospital would be affected; the sooner each department learned to function more efficiently, the better.

This consultant did what they all do - helped us administrators discover what the employer wanted us to discover. Big sheets of paper taped to the wall, magic maker words, arrows, and underlines filling the pages. Mostly, I hate this stuff. I will think I know better, and or, what is offered is not worth the time away from my primary responsibility, which I took quite seriously. I'm also not a "true believer" by which I mean I am skeptical first, before asking questions.

I went. I sat. I listened. I left at the end of the week unchanged as an administrator. In my defense, clinical engineering functions –

maintaining medical equipment – do not dove-tail neatly into other functions of a hospital, with the exceptions of the various clinical departments that use technology. What my department had to do with the fine-tuning of hospital functions, I could only guess. Turns out, I was only partially right regarding my assumptions, but almost a year would go by before I would change my view.

That year later, Larry, the director of laundry services, stopped by my office one day to chat. "Why don't you stop by and check out one of the steering committee's Friday morning meetings? You might find it interesting," he said. Likely I rolled my eyes: a meeting of corporate true believers did not sound interesting. But I liked Larry, so I did attend.

A main conference room just off the cafeteria: early Friday morning, department directors, about 30 people - there I sat coffee in hand watching and listening. The radiology department manager was obviously chairing and the conversation was open and by some appearances, honest. Friendly bunch too, so I went again next Friday, only chairing the meeting was a different person – what's going on here?

There was no chairperson, no agenda, no secretary or minutes, only participants discussing issues, not stepping on each other's sentences, not arguing or showing off. Nursing, pharmacy, security, facilities, infection control, radiology, Larry from Laundry, 15 or more, and me, discussing a wide range of issues that cut across department boundaries. Well, damn. This idea of collaboration was working, and without oversight as it turned out.

I participated for over two years until most of these administrators had changed hospitals, were laid off, or retired. On two occasions during that time, the hospital president who started this process came for a visit. In each of these instances she was asked to offer opinions on issues and each time all she said was, "Your doing fine." And she would leave. Brilliant I thought; truly empowering.

As a group, we seriously doubted this process was reproducible with any level of confidence. In fact, during an accreditation survey presentation, we were asked by a surveyor if we thought there was a formula-approach that would work to enable other hospitals to adopt our management method (whatever that was), and we all said we did not think so. Our "approach" was mostly dependent on the particular mix of people involved: How can you commodify empowerment? You can teach the idea, offer the opportunity to act independently, provide a conference room, but then you are on your own.

I became the de facto secretary, putting out a one-page newsletter each week that also served as an agenda.

Mergers, the Beginning of the End

Flying Dinosaur News

Issue No. 29　　　　**Idea Menu**　　　　October 28, 1994

☞ This Week's Agenda

Materials Management: Proposal for revised Asset Inventory Control procedures
Contract Review: Mike ▓▓▓ to give update
Job Descriptions & LOS: Lou ▓▓▓
What Is "Gentle Thursday?"

On The Left--Control Group

Below--Half Tried "Customer Relations"

Newcomers Welcome

Active Groups List

Fitness Group, #1
Standards of Behavior, #3
Utilization of Lab Tests
Standing Together, #5
Chapel Use, #5a
Pride of St. ▓▓▓, #5b
Patient Scheduling & Diagnostics
Non-Patient Transport
Lab Utilization, #7

The Steering Committee consists of managers from all departments who work on a broad range of interdisciplinary issues that contribute to quality patient care. The Steering Committee is an open forum with no chairperson and no rules. It meets once a week. All managers are welcome to attend as they see fit.
Fridays, 9 am, Travers Room 602

If you have an agenda item, please call Alan Pakaln, ext. 3118.　　"All The News That Fits"

BMET and Clinical Engineer

Flying Dinosaur News

Issue No. 28   **Idea Menu**   October 21, 1994

☞ This Week's Agenda

Materials Management: Proposal for revised Asset Inventory Control procedures.

Contract Review: Mike Mirsky to give an update.

Job Descriptions & LOS: Lou ▬▬▬

"Gentle Thursday"

Review of Minutes

MIS, Nance ▬▬▬

Maritz Report

"StoryBoard" presentation

Meeting Announcement

Waste Management, 2 PM,
Thursday, October 27, Travers 602

Active Groups List

Fitness Group, #1
Standards of Behavior, #3
Utilization of Lab Tests
Standing Together, #5
Chapel Use, #5a
Pride of St. ▬▬▬, #5b
Patient Scheduling & Diagnostics, #5c
Non-Patient Transport, #6
Lab Utilization, #7

Remember This?

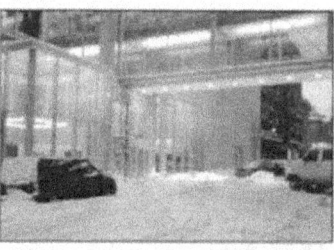

This was the scene outside the main entrance last winter after the season's biggest snowfall. The Steering Committee is taking a poll. We want to find out, on a scale of 1-10, how you rate a severe winter storm compared to preparing for the Joint Commission Survey. Come to the next meeting this Friday, and state your opinion--results next issue.

The **Flying Dinosaur Steering Committee** consists of managers from all departments who work on a broad range of interdisciplinary issues that contribute to quality patient care. The Steering Committee is an open forum with no chairperson and no rules. It meets once a week. All managers are welcome to attend as they see fit.
Fridays, 9 am, Travers Room 602

"All The News That Fits"

If you have an agenda item, please call Alan Pakaln, ext. 3118.

Mergers, the Beginning of the End

Dinosaur Article

The following are excerpts written in 1994 by three administrators, including myself, for a journal article that was never published.

> In these times of change, layoffs, bed reductions, revenue decreases, skill mix changes, and multiple other daily crises in health care, how does one create an atmosphere supportive of new ideas, new ways of thinking, new ways of approaching problem identification and problem solving in a large, urban, teaching hospital?
>
> Our institution did it with a simple children's story of a flying dinosaur and a captive group of managers who were brought together to discuss change and cost reductions. The message of the story was simple and clear : learn to fly and adapt to your surroundings, or perish. The message to the managers was clear: change to survive. If you hope to keep your job, if you want our hospital to outlive the current and coming fiscal crises in health care, if you wish to be a participant in the change, then you and your staffs had better be ready to think differently about the work environment.
>
> The initial group meetings involved 40-50 managers in one large room brainstorming as well speaking their fears about change.
>
> With each meeting, the walls were covered with detailed descriptions of what concerned the group members, what annoyed them, what they wanted to change, what they wanted to avoid, what problems did they foresee. During the following few weeks, basic common themes began to emerge that were felt to be central to the successful operation of a large teaching hospital.

A core group of managers began by holding lunchtime brown bag meetings. These would be voluntary and they decided there would be few rules to follow. There are no rules was the first. That there would be no chairperson, no one in charge, was equally important.

The participants in these first meetings were beginning to feel they had a stake in the system. The group was succeeding at more than fixing the immediate problems and promoting efficiency. They were learning new ways of working together that would carry over into other areas. The old structures were becoming old barriers and were falling.

The group was being called the Flying Dinosaurs (based on the story distributed months earlier). What are the benefits in starting or joining such a group? Lowering the walls that define and isolate departments. Creating a domain that allows people to be seen as people.

There is no formal chairperson, although the minute taker of the week has the authority to bring the group back to the subject and move the meetings along.

People grow, and become familiar with each other. This creates friendships, laughter, joy, anger, frustration, and at times, disappointment and great satisfaction.

There are risks in developing any new system of interaction. First, control must be given to those involved in order for them to take control, but most managers at our hospital reacted with hesitation more often than reckless abandon. Second, the control given up occurs inside one room for one hour a week. The Flying Dinosaurs are an addition, not a substitute. All of the original management infrastructure stay in place.

Mergers, the Beginning of the End

```
1 A Tale of Two Dinosaurs  by William
Lurcau, Quality Digest, January 1991.
2 Jeanne Marie Kiss, Ph.D.,  Senior Vice
President, Operations, St. Luke's
Division, St. Luke's-Roosevelt Hospital
Center, New York City, New York.
```

Planning by Design

Another hospital merger combined The New York Hospital, and The Presbyterian Hospital (1998). An unlikely event because each hospital was affiliated with a different, and competing, medical school: New York with Weill Cornell, and Presbyterian with Columbia University College of Physicians and Surgeons.

New job – pays much more, and all I have to so is manage the procurement of medical equipment for newly constructed facilities. I am happy, unprepared, and once again, scared that I'm ill-equipped to handle a monster job in a monster institution.

The good news was, no more 24 x 7 on-call. Much less of that kind of stress, but more adjusting to working with architects and overseeing the selection and purchase of quantities of medical equipment for newly constructed facilities. Non of which had I done previously.

How are hospital facilities, like new buildings or specialty departments created? The process is complicated, it requires specialized skills from many different disciplines all working together.

On the job training means you learn from everyone you work with. In my case I had the good fortune, and bad anxiety, to work on projects headed by a chief architect and project director.

It takes someone who has confidence, who is also charismatic in an unassuming way, and knowledgeable, and has a sensibility that includes freely expressed verbalizations (*&$#@&*!). Let's call him, Mark.

I remember the first planning meeting I attended. It was for a relatively small project, a few new procedure rooms, just basic equipment like a scale, oto-ophthalmoscope, exam light, exam table, and ancillary things like paper towel and soap dispenser, waste cans, and what's called, a sharps container for used needles.

The issues flew past me rapid fire: the number and placement of electrical outlets, splash guard for the sink, pull-curtain length, wall-mount vital signs monitor, mounted or portable? And so on. It was my first day at kindergarten, first job interview, my first day at Bellevue – all over again. I didn't know any of this stuff. For certain, I knew the equipment – that's why they hired me – but how it all fit together in a patient treatment setting, that's entirely another story. And the thing of it is, there was no reasonable way I could have expected to participate but I sure thought I should. I was knee-deep in a professional design environment, big time, and I was suppose to do something, but what was it exactly?! I felt exposed, like Rudolf with a red nose.

Creating a new medical building is an amazing thing to watch unfold. A stand-alone structure is complicated enough, but one that connects to other buildings adds anther layer of complexity. Mark chaired the weekly construction meetings that I attended, though at times you might not think anyone chaired it; most of the time, it ran itself. These meetings were attended by construction supervisors, architects, a hospital administrator,

Depending on the scale of a project, many different kinds of people can participate in various kinds of planning meetings: administrators, nurses, doctors, architects, other department representatives like housekeeping, infection control, a construction management. Regular planning meetings occur at the very beginning of a project where the scope of services are discussed right through to the end as the punch list is resolved.

Meetings can be tense where an "outside" opinion becomes a challenge to authority: A vice president presents a design for the efficient transfer of patients to a unit when the housekeeping manager questions how collected waste can be stored for the end-of-day pickup in that same hallway where patients are waiting for a room. All eyes are on the challenger and everyone is waiting for the VP response.

Hospital atmosphere can be supportive and encourage challenges, or they can become contentious because the meeting chair has something personal to prove and will not surrender any authority. I have worked in both. But it can be a tough choice as some "authorities" actually are just that, and too much discussion can lead to chaos, which if allowed to continue can ruin a project. Challengers must learn from experience to choose battles; decide

Mergers, the Beginning of the End

when to learn and from whom.

Leadership needs to be sensitive enough to know when to protect the challengers, but leaders can have negative consequences for a challenger, even if the action is followed.

Not being a team player can be interpreted many different ways

In the eight years I worked at New York Presbyterian, I witnessed the second in command be replaced, and both the medical director of the emergency department and the head nurse fired. Exactly why these people were fired I do not know. In my limited capacity, I enjoyed working with them and thought they did a great job. Obviously I did not see everything they did, but my point here is that I suspect the larger and the more aggressive an institution is, the greater the pressure is to outperform the status quo. In an institution less concerned with a national rating, any of these people may have shined.

Today, everything is more competitive so it's not surprising that hospitals compete for patients. How hospitals compete is a complicated issue, but significant ones are proficiency in an treatment area, and outcomes: do a lot of hip replacements and have great results, and you may get more business. Do this, with as few available beds as possible: it keeps expenses for the hospital down, and lower bed numbers acts as an incentive for hospitals to keep admissions down – lower admissions means lower Medicare/Medicaid federal reimbursements.

Consequently, many states require justification and detailed plans to be submitted for any expansion approvals. And just creating those justifications costs money – which drives up costs overall.

Among the costs that can increase with time are loan guarantees. I have worked on projects that were rushed somewhat in order to meet financing deadlines. Projects are also rushed to meet supply contract prices as well as competing with another hospital for a similar new patient service. In that sense, medicine is just like any other business.

BMET and Clinical Engineer

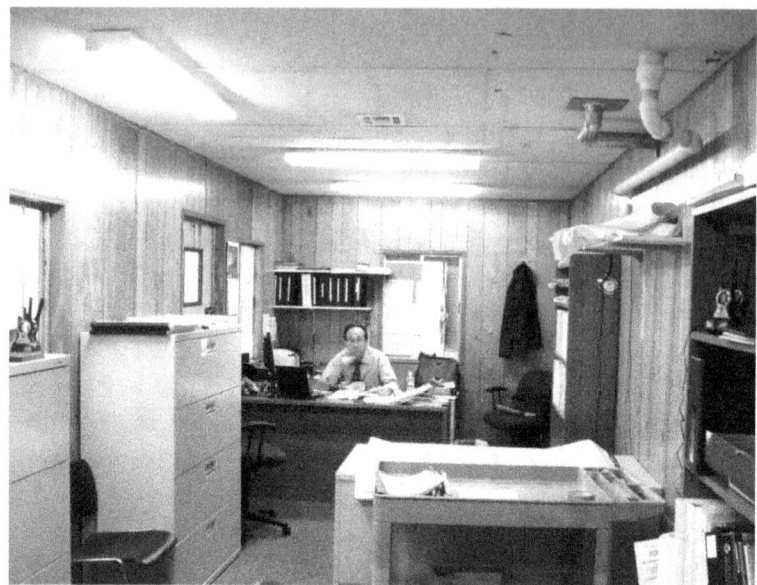

Office in a temporary trailer. Three of us were hired to purchase the medical equipment for the New York-Presbyterian Heart Center.

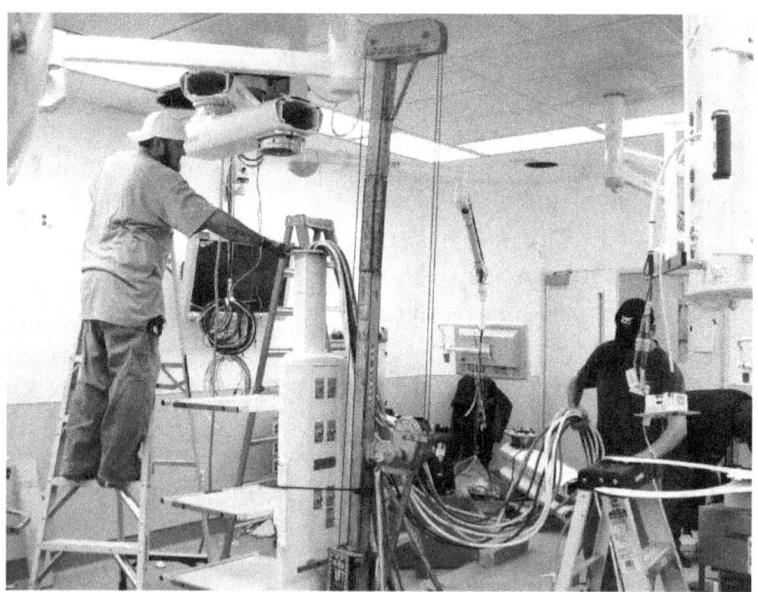

OR Installation

Risky Business

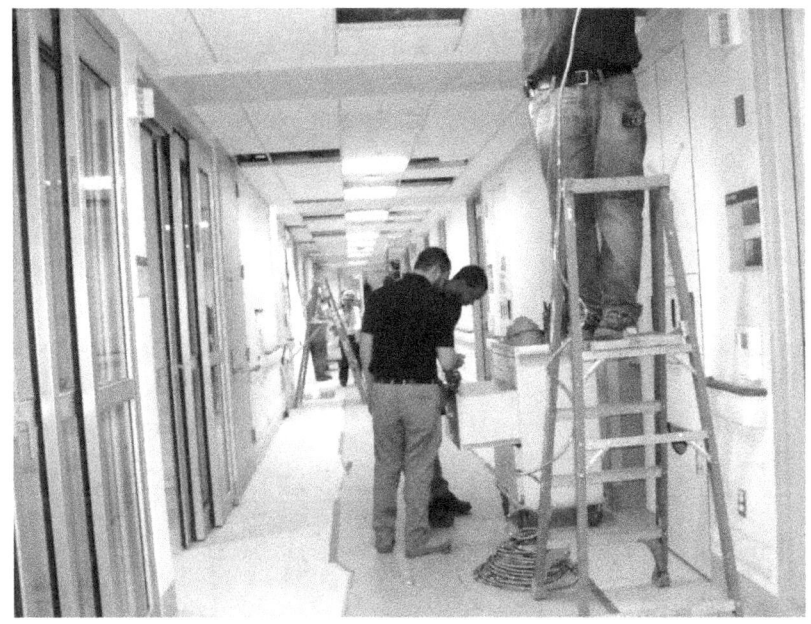

NY Presbyterian Hospital, new construction.

BMET and Clinical Engineer

I think that in terms of how most of us live our lives – myself include – we will at times be just plain stupid when it comes to assessing risk, predicting that the results of our actions will be much more or much less risky than desirable. I am referring to the many different kinds of decisions we might make - maybe the car we buy, or how we ride a bike, eat, house ourselves, insure ourselves, medicate or inoculate ourselves, or save money. Most of us have a narrow view of, not whether there *may be* risks, but of how we might go about assessing the risk-odds, should we wish to.

I am not opposed to the idea of playing dare-devil if that's your cup of tea, however missing a way to assess risk and proceeding blindly in addressing that risk, only narrows ones options. We are left to relying only on our own predispositions, which can leave us falling short of a canyon edge so to speak (Evel Knievel's son made the Grand Canyon jump in 1999).

For hospitals, nursing homes, and outpatient clinics - the facilities that are accredited - risk assessment begins with cost savings, and ends with accreditation. That is, all institutions start their fiscal year with a planned budget, and from there, determine the best rout to satisfying accreditation standards.

Other than setting program standards in order to cause no harm to a patient, the primary motivation for assessing risk is to create efficient services. It's a practical decision. Otherwise, having no concern for cost could conceivably place a nurse and doctor at every bedside 24 x 7, just in case. A line <u>must</u> be drawn somewhere, somehow; risk assessment is the how.

Assessing risk is a *reasoned* process that ends with the adoption of standards of care, balancing the minimum possible (cost-saving) care with the lowest possibility of causing harm. In other words, get the job done with the least cost, but in a way that avoids harm to the patient. Once this balance has been achieved, the appropriate clinical administrator then writes a policy that spells out, in detail: the necessary procedures to follow, and the staff education to back it up.

The risk assessment process generates a standard when the risk is identified and procedures are developed to reduce that risk. The risk assessment process is at the foundation of the many functions prescribed in hospitals - the committees, policies and procedures, and standards, all reflect that process. That's the chain: from risk to accreditation.

Admit it, you'd rather guess

As for us humans, assessing risk in life is the elephant in the room - something important, very obvious, and actively avoided. Generally speaking, we'd rather sit back and modify our behavior according to our own inclination than do the homework of assessing actual risk: won't get on that plane, but I will finish my golf game even though I hear thunder.

For many assessments of risk, we take for granted that someone is doing the job correctly and everything is being taken care of, like the break job on your car, food you buy at the market, or the plane ride – experts have looked things over and have determined the best coarse of action.

If you're looking for trouble, you're looking at risk

Almost everyone working at a job is assigned a specific function, and if while performing that function, something needs to be done, it should get done. Or it gets called in for someone else's job function to address. Let's say everyone working in your local hospital is doing their job exactly the way they should be doing it; 100% perfect, A+. Is that enough? Are hospital staff really doing *everything* that needs to be done?

Your answer to this question – based on real life experience - should be: Probably not. Because in real life, things can almost always be improved. And besides, mistakes happen, or things just get left off the to-do list and everyone just keeps driving over the same pothole that never gets fixed.

Everyone working in a hospital has a specific function: housekeepers clean, doctors do doctoring; nurses nursing, cooks cook, and phlebotomists draw blood. But is anyone going around just looking for things that got "left off the to-do list?" At this point, I can hear medical staff responding: "Yes there are people doing this! Administrators walk around all the time looking for issues needing resolution."

There are quality reviews, and problem-solving meetings; lots of meetings. And all staff are regularly trained to be diligent in observing and reporting problems: We run a tight ship! It's true, hospitals are sensitive about their reputations and they dedicate resources that address safety and efficacy. The thing is, that while room cleaning, medical treatments, vital signs taking, nutrition, and blood draws, all can be observed, assessed, and results trended and reported through meetings and follow-up emails, these are all specific functions that attract focused and directed attention. Meanwhile, technology is everywhere, embedded in many things, increasing the possibility that something nefarious can be missed.

Hospitals depend on staff to call attention to sloppy behavior or failed devices. Here, from my experience, are some of the possibilities when everyday life intervenes.

- The note says, "BROKEN." It's stuck on a device and left in a corner to be found, or not.
- An EKG machine is thrown down a fire escape stairwell, no note.
- Found in a closet, dusty, dirty, and broken.
- Message on department service phone line: "Seven North: a monitor doesn't work. Thanks." Who? Which? What?
- Equipment cart found outside the service shop door, no note.

When it comes to technology, staff are trained to see and act within their own sphere, their own realm. With one possible exception: the CE staff. They can act like the local police and walk around patrolling, looking for the defective plug on a patient bed, the defective IV pump hidden in a closet, or the dirty lens on a wall ophthalmoscope (The thing clinicians use to look at your retina; lens cleaning can go unchecked).

Medical errors kill and maim patients, but so does defective technology, and so does inattention. Having someone assigned to go out looking for problems is a good idea.

Here I can speak from personal experience.

Overseeing the day-to-day operations servicing any and all the medical technology in large hospitals, I was able to address the issue of operational oversight in two ways: 1. I could assign a CE technician to perform scheduled "area inspections." Which were just that: The technician walks around, looking in all the hiding places, speaking with staff, and taking notes regarding rumors, first-hand accounts, and complaints. 2. I would walk around doing the same thing.

Clinical staff have a "funny" relationship with medical technology: some love it, but many — just like anywhere else - are intimidated by it, and some avoid it as much as possible. Having a technology-oriented person - a BMET or CE - walk around the institution making personal contact with staff can have a reassuring effect. It also promotes good will, which can translate into better reporting and more frequent questions being asked, which in tern, can translate into better use of technology and better treatment of patients.

Improving relationships with staff and their use of technology sounds like a good idea, doesn't it? Can the medical industry promote this? Should it be a part of a hospital accreditation? Is there a way to institutionalize the process of personalizing oversight? The short answer is, yes. The long answer is, it depends on the structure and personal makeup of the particular hospital organization (Even though the Flying Dinosaur group succeeded at one hospital, St. Luke's, and managers worked at both merged facilities, there was universal skepticism that a similar group could work at the other hospital).

The job of maintaining medical equipment and associated technology in hospitals has matured: it now comes in one of two basic forms: for-profit business, and the more traditional department, owned and operated by a hospital. There are real incentives to outsourcing equipment service: there is a potential for medical facilities to save money, and outsourcing takes the worry out of understanding the technology. If you think keeping track of all the consumer electronic gadgets can be intimidating, it does not begin to compare with the issues medical technology can present.

As a cost-savings potential, outsourcing - as many businesses realize - can go this way or that way, depending on many variables. Larger institutions may be able to negotiate service that offers the possibility of saving money. But then, after some time, discover either that service is lacking, or safety issues offer a compelling argument to run their own department. Which is why institutions will switch, back and forth, depending on who the institution's safety officer or bean-counter is at the time.

What challenges does an institution take on in managing their

own in-house medical technology service? Lots. There are some shared responsibilities with other departments, but generally, here is a list of what a service department can be responsible for:
- Medical equipment repair.
- Budget and service contract oversight.
- Accreditation survey preparation.
- Failure and safety issue reporting.
- Risk management and periodic maintenance.

Who oversees whom?

Departments have directors; department directors report to administrators; administration has to comply with survey standards, state and accreditation; accreditation surveyors report to their accreditation organization. Who watches the accreditation organizations? Right answer: the CMS, Centers for Medicare and Medicaid Services. Who watches the CMS is another story; more on that later.

Hospital-run departments require administrative oversight. And while there are several hospital administration jobs that are not very user-friendly, this is definitely one of them. Here are two reasons why: 1. Technology is always changing, and not in the direction of becoming less complicated. Or less competitive: deciding on vendors based mainly on price is not usually possible to do. 2. Budget approval: you must constantly compare outsourcing the thingamajig machine with in-house service. And you must justify the money you spend on preventive maintenance – how do you sell the possibility that you avoided catastrophe, when you can not prove that catastrophe would happen?

Preventive maintenance requires staff, and staff are FTEs (full time employees), that last thing a hospital wants to spend money on because it is on-going. Paying money to avoid risk is one of the most difficult argument to win. But when failure and injury occurs, you can be sure every single decision you made will be scrutinized. This is a very good argument for a risk management program, and a rationale that can be explained and understood.

If an institution manages its own service, or maintains a close administrative relationship with a service provider, that institution may be able to excel at providing a safer treatment environment – safer than institutions that sign away oversight with little involvement in that oversight.

In other words, CE technicians in a hospital may be empowered and incentivized to actively look for problems, or not. It all depends on who is supervising, and who is supervising the supervisors.

Basic risk assessment

Risk assessment is not "rocket science." Actually it is partly, but as for the expression, it does not have to be very complicated. It is a reasoned and disciplined approach to better understanding risk and more easily see how one proposed solution compares with another. The process is often described as comparing, benefit to risk.

The steps are relatively simple.

Clearly state the issue and the risks – the potential to cause harm.

Describe ways in which those risks can be reduced.

Decide if the benefits you get from reducing risks are enough to warrant making an adjustment.

Document the results.

Generally speaking, the assessment of risk is comprised of two things: the degree of harm or loss that may occur, and the likelihood of that harm occurring. Risk factors are the specific things that the risk is made of: if crossing the street is the risk being assessed, where you cross, and the number and speed of vehicles, are the risk factors.

The Basic Idea

Degree of Harm	Likelihood of Harm Happening		
	High	Med	Low
High	High Priority	High Priority	Med Priority
Med	High Priority	Med Priority	Low Priority
Low	Med Priority	Low Priority	Low Priority

Looked at together, they can form a matrix that effectively offers a rating. Added to other details of an issue produces the risk-to-benefit outcome. The following is a screen-shot of a program that manages the information used in making assessments that determine how periodic (preventive) maintenance is performed.

Risky Business

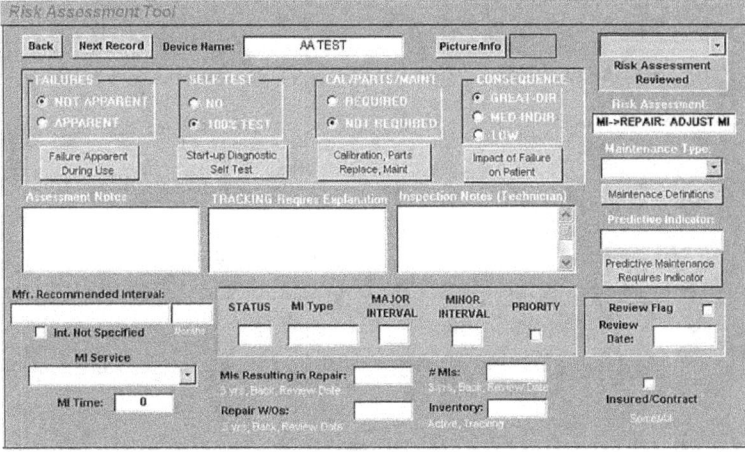

The process of risk assessment is discussed and debated in professional journals and within various related organizations such as The Joint Commission. The center of much of this debate concerns the relationships of service data to risk. Additional service data includes such things as failure and repair frequency, life-support functions, and the ability of a device operator to detect a failure before it affects the patient.

While the general notion of risk – the basic matrix – is well understood and accepted, the process of integrating all the variables and generating a result, is not. It is mainly for this reason that there is no standard for how hospitals assess risk nor how hospitals establish their maintenance schedule.

BMET and Clinical Engineer

Improvements

Over time, medical technology gets better; thee are fewer failures due to design and manufacturing faults, while at the same time, much of technology becomes more complicated, to make and to use.

Infant Incubators

Used in NICU, early models had a water reservoir with a fan blowing air across to humidify the air, important for developing lungs.

The problem was these pools of water were also breeding bacteria and infecting new-borns.

During this same early period, mercury thermometers were also in use, and broken ones would make their way into the reservoirs below the bed – air from the fans picked up evaporating mercury (the way liquid mercury can be absorbed) and fed to the infant.

BMET and Clinical Engineer

Trying to Make Things Better

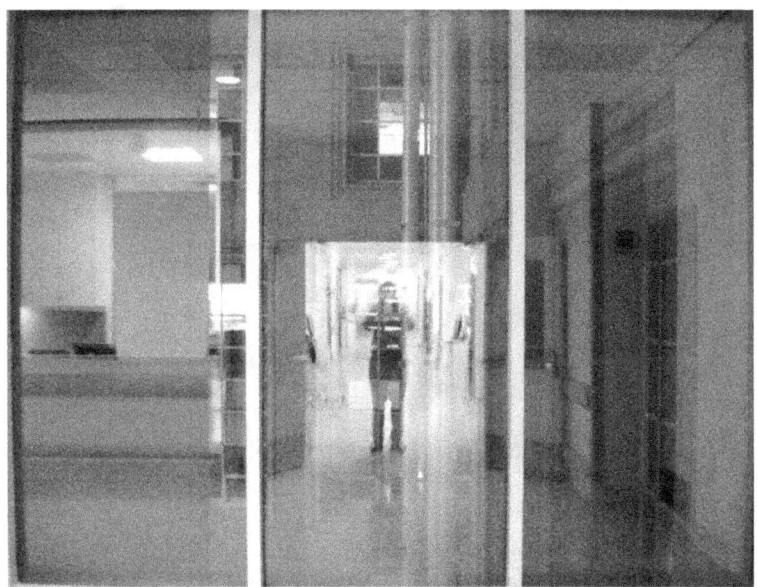

Alone in a new unopened building (NYP Heart Center),
just walking around reflecting on the job.

BMET and Clinical Engineer

*M*edical practice standards are developed by a range of organizations — federal state government, nonprofit and for-profit - in what is called a self-regulated industry. In this case it means that the main overseer — the federal government — places trust in the relevant organizations to manage themselves. This makes sense because, for example, the organizations that survey hospitals to be accredited presumably know much more about the details of medical practice than a bureaucrat "sitting in Washington."

On the other hand, as they say on the farm, who is watching over the henhouse? The farmer, or the rooster? Not the best analogy. The real question - and it is not an easy one to answer – is, who besides medical experts checks to make sure the medical experts are not making things just a little bit too easy for themselves?

The actual answer is, the Centers for Medicare & Medicaid Services (CMS) is where the "buck stops," where the "rubber meets the road," where the money is: if a hospital wants to receive Medicare reimbursements, it must be accredited – to be accredited, it must pass survey inspections from at least one of four survey organizations. And to pass survey a medical treatment facility must satisfy prescribed standards, standards set by the survey organization and approved by the CMS.

Hospitals, nursing homes, ambulatory care centers pay to be surveyed, and to some extent, the four survey organizations are competing for business from these groups. The four survey organizations must convince the CMS that they are providing a viable service in how they accredit, at the same time, there is incentive for the four to make the certification process acceptable to treatment facilities. In other words, it is to everyone's advantage – hospitals, the four survey organizations, and the CMS – to find methods that make everyone look good. In plain English.

The path to assessing the risks of medical technology – its procedures and machines - and the application of standards, is a fuzzy one because there is no one kind of machine with easy-to-define characteristics, and because machines often function in a close partnership with clinicians.

Accreditation

There are a total of 6,210 hospital facilities in the U.S. (2019). Of these, 4,773 are registered with the CMS, which means they subscribe to one of the four accreditation organizations and are surveyed. Hospitals are required to adhere to state health department regulations, but they are not required by law to participate in accreditation surveys. Most do, however, in order to satisfy federal requirements for accepting Medicare or Medicaid payments.

The purpose of an accreditation survey is two-fold: To assure specific quality standards are met, and in theory at least, to act as an educational platform for learning how to do things better. In order to appreciate how these standards function it would help to first understand certain unique issues.

There are fundamental differences between how medical technology is managed and overseen and how the rest of medicine functions, at least in terms of how risks are managed. Physicians often explain the risks inherent in a procedure, but rating risks for technology is rarely a clear path. As it was in this example.

A 2004 FDA rule mandated the use of medication barcodes as part of a patient's wristband. This rule was passed in order to address the potential for a wrong medication to be administered to a patient. This idea is fairly easy to understand and appreciate: To help reduce medication errors by humans, use a certified machine program to oversee matching medication to patient instead of an error-prone human.

The FDA mandates a new regulation, and CMS, with assistance from various organizations and perhaps hospitals, writes a standard and pushes it out to all medical facilities. Those facilities' administrators then write policies that are specific for different departments: Nurses may have procedures different from doctors, and different from pharmacy – but all must satisfy the regulation as stated by the CMS.

How risks are assessed for medical equipment failures is quite another story.

The CMS has approved four organizations to set standards, survey, and accredit healthcare facilities like hospitals, nursing homes, ambulatory care centers. Three of the four are nonprofit organizations: Healthcare Facilities Accreditation Program (HFAP),

Center for Improvement in Healthcare Quality (CIHQ), The Joint Commission (TJC). One is a for-profit company, a branch of a large multinational, DNV GL Healthcare.

Of these four, The Joint Commission is arguably the largest. TJC surveys nearly 21,000 healthcare organizations, hospitals, nursing homes, etc. Their stated mission is, "To continuously improve health care for the public." As in all industries, since its beginning in 1951 TJC standards have been evolving; part of their stated purpose is to research and educate.

All of these organizations' survey methods require approval by the CMS. CMS a BIG organization and their website is not a simple one. After all, it provides information to a lot of people who use their services - those over age 65 for starters. Their mission states: "CMS must ensure that these individuals (90 million Americans) have access to high quality care."

The development of standards is a complicated process: there are many medical specialties, each with their own unique characteristics requiring a nuanced understanding. Standards will often require interpretation by a range of experts in various fields. Nothing is simple when it comes to standards and oversight.

Here's how the system for hospital medical equipment standards works.

The CMS sets a standard, in broad terms. This standard states that hospitals must "ensure an acceptable level of safety and quality" (42 CFR Ch. IV (10–1–18 Edition: § 482.41). Then organizations in the business of quality assurance develop the working standards for hospitals and submit them to CMS for approval. The four organizations approved to accredit hospitals by the CMS are: Healthcare Facilities Accreditation Program (HFAP), Center for Improvement in Healthcare Quality (CIHQ), DNV GL - Healthcare (DNV GL), and The Joint Commission (TJC).

The interpretation of standards is not as well defined as one might think, and actually makes use of inputs from organizations like the Association for the Advancement of Medical Instrumentation (AAMI), the American Society for Health Care Engineering of the American Hospital Association (ASHE), and even the National Fire Protection Association (NFPA).

Healthcare services in the U.S. are self-regulated, and someone must foot the cost of paying those standard writers and surveyors salaries. Hospitals pay to be surveyed for accreditation, and the accreditation organizations compete for a hospital's business.

The process of having the same organizations that are responsible for assessing accreditation standards – HFAP, CIHQ, DNV GL, TJC – also being the source of those standards, could be seen as a conflict of interest. Especially when you consider that offering a standard that is easier for a hospital to meet could have a greater appeal than one that is harder to meet.

Standards vs. interpretation

The fact that standards are only truly established once they have been interpreted is the single most important issue impacting the maintenance oversight of medical equipment. It is important because requiring the interpretation of standards then necessitates the interpretation of what it means to be in compliance. The CMS began their efforts overseeing medical equipment maintenance by establishing the #1 rule: "Medical equipment must be inspected periodically." That became the standard for hospital accreditation.

The actual history of this rule and policy will show this simple policy alongside institutional responses: "Wait. Inspect what equipment, ALL equipment? That would be an inefficient use of resources – not all medical equipment needs periodic inspecting. Like a simple exam light - anyone can see if the light doesn't work, and when it doesn't, we have the light replaced." Fair enough.

So each hospital was told to come up with its own rationale for what equipment is in, and which is out. Over time, this piece of the maintenance standard evolved and changed to incorporate a range of criteria that would determine inclusion in a maintenance program. For example, life support equipment must be inspected, and with a relatively short inspection interval. This is where risk assessment procedures, and the different types of medical facilities would impact oversight standards.

The CMS along with the four approved survey organizations are overseeing a very large group of different kinds of medical services, everything from outpatient clinics and nursing homes, to networks of hospitals. Among the survey organizations there were stated concerns that establishing one policy that defines exactly what and how medical equipment is inspected could work for some facilities but not for others.

The CMS could accept unique policies for unique facilities assuming surveyors could come up with a workable standard that promoted safety and quality care at all facilities, while allowing for different approaches.

This variance was a critical turning point in how standards were going to be set. And, unfortunately, it allowed for some forms of dissociated data management and skewed record keeping.

What exactly were those facility differences that resulted in different standards to be set for different medical facilities? Was it to accommodate different economic circumstances? Training problems? Political push-back from the now huge and formidable medical institutions?

A similar situation: the airline industry

One way to explain the situation medical facilities are in is to use oversight of the airline industry as an example. Just like hospitals, each plane is different, each manufacturer has a different style of management.

The FAA is mandated to be the expert of all that. It's very hard to do, so they delegate.

According to the Federal Aviation Administration (FAA), their mission is: to provide the safest, most efficient aerospace system in the world." Zowee, both *safe* and *efficient* (Sounds like a potential conflict of interest to me). And there have been problems - as we have learned – when the FAA assigns authority to aircraft manufacturers with minimum oversight.

It has recently been made clear that the Federal Aviation Administration (FAA) merely reviews detailed analysis concerning safe (low risk) construction of aircraft, rather than performing their own analysis, or the direct oversight of a manufacturer's. Risk assessment takes time, work, and experts, all of which costs money.

This is not entirely unreasonable. Aircraft companies already have the knowledge base and the experience to perform comprehensive assessments, hence the efficient cost-saving FAA decision to let them do the work. This works except when details are missed, and assessments are incomplete (and people die).

Consider this: How comfortable would you feel flying if the

airline industry announced that maintenance inspections on aircraft would be tracked by how often technicians report to work on time – instead of tracking the numbers of aircraft actually inspected? This is how compliance rates are set for the periodic maintenance of medical equipment in hospitals and nursing homes: Inspections are tracked by rates of adherence to a schedule, not by the count of equipment actually inspected.

I tried

According to the Agency for Healthcare Research and Quality (AHRQ), there are 88 federally listed organizations dedicated to patient safety in the United States. Searching "patient safety" in Amazon.com books returns over 2,000, in Google search, 23,300,000 results (2020). As to tracking problems, the federal government maintains a database of malpractice reports. Hospitals have access to these reports, but most individuals and the general public do not ("The reports are confidential, and not available to the public.") There are nonprofit organizations that work with the FDA and the CMS. For medical technology, three of the larger are the Emergency Care Research Institute (ECRI), the Association for the Advancement of Medical Instrumentation (AAMI), and U.S. Pharmacopeia.

It seems to me that if you are in the "business" of trying to make things better, at some point you have felt alone in your efforts. That at the least, the line of people at your door waiting to help you in your cause is short. It's often a hard road just getting anyone's attention, the media-scape is so full. But, by all indications, there are in fact a lot of people trying to make things better. And I am one of them.

For about two years, during 2018-2019, I contacted – by letter post, and email - over 800 medical safety officers, MDs, and journalists in an effort to spread the word regarding the crazy way in which compliance is calculated in this country. Actually, first I engaged in email discussions, if you can call them that, with administrators at TJC. I did this twice over a period of several decades. I also engaged in discussions and wrote two peer-reviewed journal articles, one about compliance calculations, published in AAMI, one of several organizations who help set accreditation standards. Crazy, right? Crazy because only a handful responded and

Trying to Make Things Better

yet I continued.

Disappointed is the word. And the reason to continue pursuing an issue even when your efforts produce no tangible results is – just to do it, not for the success, but for the practice of working towards something you believe in. But, maybe my not succeeding in getting my message across has been due to one or more of the following:

- My message is wrong; there really is no problem to begin with.
- I'm not very good at explaining the issue.
- Compliance calculation does not have the attraction of a new app, or Netflix series, or news flash: it is difficult to explain in a way that makes it easy to comprehend; it takes effort to understand it.
- People are busy, and in the field of medicine, directed to more urgent hazards. Of which there are many.

But let's say – as a few MD safety officers did – you do understand and appreciate the issue of maintenance compliance and how it could adversely affect patient care, then what? How does one cause change in such a huge and bureaucratic system as healthcare represents?

It's a tough question because:

- There are four certification groups, each with their own methods.
- These four groups are in fact competing with each other for the business that medical facilities represent – charging to survey is how survey groups survive, and how attractive their survey is to a hospital (how easy they can pass?) can make one survey group better off financially.
- The CMS, though assigned the responsibility of oversight, in actuality, relies on the certification groups. So forget about appealing the CMS, it's the four survey groups you must approach.

And the four survey groups already have developed methods that let hospitals, nursing homes, and urgent care centers look good as they adhere to standards – there just is no incentive to make things more difficult than they already are. Compliance calculation just opens up the proverbial can of worms. Ick! Who likes worms?

BMET and Clinical Engineer

It's Not a Fun Subject

`It's not a fun subject.`

No sexy alarmist headlines to see, no Tweets or Facebook Likes: YOUR HOSPITAL EQUIPMENT MAINTENANCE IS ON SCHEDULE AND OUT OF DATE!

But this is true for many healthcare institutions.

Hospitals reporting 100% compliant are probably not inspecting all their medical equipment on time.

Actually, inspecting equipment 100% on time is almost impossible to achieve.

The accreditation standard is to follow a *schedule of inspections* 100% of the time.

Therefor hospitals can report 100% completion rates and be "compliant."

Results: Patients can be put at risk. And no one knows what the actual inspection completion rates of equipment - they know the rates of adhering to a schedule, but not of the number of devices inspected.

Put another way:

What do you think the reaction would be if the airline industry announced that maintenance inspections on aircraft would be tracked by how often technicians report to work on time — instead of tracking the numbers of aircraft actually inspected? The obvious answer is there would be some sort of intense reaction to this news. However, this is exactly how the Joint Commission rates compliance for the periodic maintenance of medical equipment.

Of the 21,000 Joint Commission surveyed institutions, no one knows the inspection rate for medical equipment – not despite Joint standards, but because of them. This fact represents possible patient safety issues, but because there is no data, no one knows how this plays out in terms of reported incidents: incidents must be reported, but actual maintenance compliance is not.

How is this possible?

The Joint Commission accreditation standard for medical equipment maintenance is 100%. However, inspecting 100% of the medical equipment on time is not just difficult for many institutions, it is virtually impossible to achieve because some equipment invariably is "missing" during inspections: "floaters" like IV pumps travel from one department to another, equipment may be stolen or transferred to another department, rentals are returned, staff may hide equipment because of perceived shortages, a department may send something out for repair, equipment can be in use on a patient, or perhaps maintenance technicians are just not as thorough as they might be.

The policy

The Joint does not require 100% of the equipment to be inspected on time.

Their policy requires that maintenance technicians follow an inspection schedule 100% of the time. However a technician can adhere to a schedule regardless of the number of equipment pieces that are inspected: miss some equipment in a scheduled location, you can just move on to the next scheduled location.

It is understandable how technicians can be motivated to stay on schedule to avoid being cited on a survey.

It's Not a Fun Subject

A Problem

Equipment not inspected can be "missing" or just not looked for during the prescribed inspection period. "Missing" equipment does not become part of the compliance calculation and reporting, even though some of the uninspected equipment may be in use on patients.

Why would The Joint set a standard of 100%, when it is virtually impossible to inspect all equipment 100% on time?

1. 100% means The Joint does not need to justify setting a standard anything lower (more realistic), e.g. 95%. What science could they use in their rationale?

2. The Joint can have just one standard for everyone: smaller facilities (with lower numbers of "missing" equipment), and larger facilities (with higher numbers of "missing" equipment). One standard for all, instead of two, needs no explanation.

The reason this standard is bad

No one can tell from compliance reporting what the actual level of equipment inspections is, nor can anyone see how long some equipment remains uninspected. Also, less meaningful data means less diligence: what incentive to improve is there if you can always achieve 100%, even when you are not?

A Proposed Fix

First, show real numbers so everyone can know what the actual rate of inspected equipment is. If the rate is 95%, state that, and state why it is 95% and not higher. Second, show the percent and breakdown of equipment not located ("missing"). If the inspection rate is 95%, explain the 5% so that everyone can assess the quality of inventory (a side benefit), and more clearly track and focus on what is not inspected and why it isn't.

Periodic compliance reporting should look something like this: using a total inventory quantity of 1,000 with 95% of inventory inspected on time, the remaining 5%, or 50 pieces, are past due. This uninspected or unlocated equipment should be explained – e.g., in shop, on patient, or other – along with numbers of intervals missed. The uninspected or unlocated equipment consists of the following:

BMET and Clinical Engineer

# Intervals Missed	Equipment Qty	Exception/Reason	Notes
1	13	In service shop	
1	10	In use on patient	
2	9	Did not locate	
3	6	Did not locate	
4	4	Did not locate	
5	3	Did not locate	
>5	5	Did not locate	Remove 4 from inventory
Totals:	50		

And of course, at some point, equipment that is not located for some prescribed period can be removed from inventory – after findings are reported, reviewed and signed off by various personnel.

The cutoff from compliance calculation, as shown here, is 18 months. The greatest area under the curve represents the 95% of inventory in compliance. Between the "date of compliance calculation" and the 18 month cutoff is the 5% of inventory that is

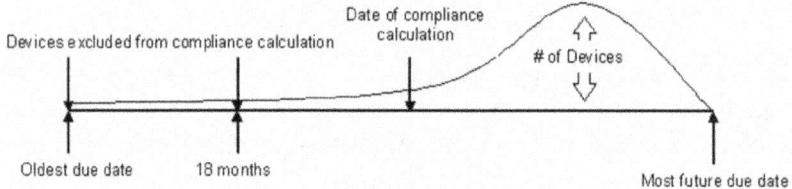

out of date. Between the 18 month cutoff and "oldest due date" is removed from calculation, but still reported.

A standard

What policy can The Joint Commission establish to promote maintenance safety, and be appropriate to all? If The Joint had been collecting real data for a period of time, perhaps a meaningful percent could now be set as a standard, tailored for different institution types and sizes. But as things stand now, meeting a standard must mean you meet or better the institution's benchmark: e.g. 95% compliant with 5% uninspected or missing, means that the institution must meet or better those numbers in the next survey. Or satisfactorily explain why it can't.

Real maintenance compliance numbers, trended over time, will place a clearer focus on the efforts made to improve performance. Real numbers measure actual results, and the surveyor always has the prerogative of accepting explanations for numbers that deviate from the norm.

The proposed fix keeps the issue of unlocated inventory front and center where it should be. What incentive is there to improve if – as is the case now – you rely on a system that all but guarantees 100%? When it's likely you are not.

What you don't know can hurt.

Every medical facility will have its own way of classifying devices, there is no standard. The following was used in one of the hospitals I worked in.

BMET and Clinical Engineer

Col1	Col2	Col3	Col4	Col5	Col6
ABSORBER, ANES	CHEST X-RAY	ERGOMETER	LASER, MULTIWAVE	OTO/OPHTH MOBILE	SEQUENTIAL COMP, FOOT
ACQUISITION MODULE	CINE PROJECTOR	ESU	LASER, UV	OTO/OPHTH SCOPE TRAN	SEQUENTIAL COMP, LEG
AERATOR	CLOCK/RADIO	ESU, LOW POWER	LASER, YAG	OXIMETER FINGERPROBE	SHAKER, LABORATORY
AIR FRESHENER	CLOCK/TIMER	EVACUATION HOOD	LATHE, DENTAL	OXIMETER, PULSE	SIMULATOR, PATIENT
ALARM, NON MEDICAL	CODE ZERO ALARM	EXERCISER, BICYCLE	LENSOMETER	OXIMETER, PULSE, 515 B	SIREN/PA
ALARM, REMOTE	COLD LIGHT HARDENER	EXERCISER, ELBOW	LESION GENERATOR	OXIMETER, PULSE, ANES	SLIDE COVER MACHINE
AMPLIFIER, AUDIO	COLD PACK UNIT	EXERCISER, LEG	LIFT, PATIENT	OXIMETER, PULSE/CAPNO	SLIDE VIEWER
ANALYZER, PLASMA PRO	COLPOSCOPE	FAIL-SAFE MONITOR	LIGHT SOURCE	OXIMETER, WHOLE BLOOD	SLIT LAMP
ANALYZER, BLOOD COAG	COMPRESSOR, AIR	PAX	LIGHT SOURCE TRANSF	OXYGEN CONCENTRATOR	SLUSH UNIT
ANALYZER, BLOOD GAS	COMPRESSOR/ASPIRATOR	FETAL HEART DET, US	LIGHT, EXAMINATION	OXYGEN MONITOR	SPHYG, ANEROID
ANALYZER, CHEMISTRY	COMPUTER	FIBRILLATOR	LIGHT, PROCEDURE, DERM	OXYGEN MONITOR, ANES	SPIROMETER
ANALYZER, CO	COMPUTER, ARRHYTHMIA	FILM PROCESSOR	LIGHT, SURGICAL, OR	PA SYSTEM	STADIOMETER
ANALYZER, DNA	COMPUTER, PC	FILM VIEWER	LINE ISOLATION MON	PACE CARD ESOPHAGEAL	STAINER, SLIDE
ANALYZER, EAR	COMPUTER, US IMAGER	FILTER, AIR	LITHOTRITE	PACE CARD EX INVASE	STAINER, ELECTRIC
ANALYZER, GAS, ANES	CONSOLE, THERMO	FILTER, AIR/UV	MAMMOGRAPHY X-RAY	PACE PROGRAMMER	STAPLER, SURGICAL
ANALYZER, GLUCOSE	CONTROLLER, BIPAP	FILTER, TANK, METABOL	MAMMOGRAPHY, DIGITAL	PACE, NONVASE, DEFIB	STEREOTACTIC SURG SY
ANALYZER, HEPARIN	CONTROLLER, DRILL, IRR	FIRE ALARM SYSTEM	MANOMETER, ANEROID	PACEMAKER ANALYZER	STERILIZER, CHEMICAL
ANALYZER, METABOLIC	CONTROLLER, DRILL, SUR	FLOURESCEIN ANGIO	MANOMETER, PULMONARY	PACKAGE SEALER	STERILIZER, DENT
ANALYZER, OXYGEN	CONTROLLER, MULTIPORT	FLOWMETER, ULTRASONIC	MEDICATION DISPENSER	PARALLEL BARS	STERILIZER, GAS
ANALYZER, TISSUE	CONTROLLER, SHAVER	FLUID-GAS EXCHANGER	METER, DIGITAL PRESS	PERFUSION SYSTEM	STERILIZER, PLASMA
ANALYZER, URINE	CONTROLLER, TEMP	FLUIDOTHERAPY UNIT	METER, POSTAL	PH METER	STERILIZER, STEAM
ANESTHESIA MACHINE	CONTROLLER, VIDEO	FLUOROSCOPY SYSTEM	METER, POT ACUITY	PHOTOTACHOMETER	STILL, VAPONICS
ANGIOGRAPHY SYSTEM	COUNTER, GAMMA	FLUROCOUNT	MICROFILM READER	PHOTOTHERAPY UNIT	STIMULATOR, NEUROMUSC
ANGIOPLASTY, ROTATION	COUNTER, SCINTALLATIO	FOOT SWITCH	MICROSCOPE, LAB	PLETHYSMOGRAPH	TABLE, EXAMINATION
APHERESIS UNIT	CRANIOTOME, MOTOR ASY	FREEZER, PLASMA	MICROSCOPE, LAB, LIGHT	PORTABLE X-RAY	TABLE, OPERATING
ARTH SURG PWR UNIT	CRYOCONSOLE	GAMMA CAMERA	MICROSCOPE, OPERATING	POSITIONING GUIDE	TABLE, PHYS THERAPY
ARTHROSCOPIC SYSTEM	CRYO-PRESERVATION	GAMMA CAMERA, MOBILE	MIDDLE EAR ANALYZER	POWER SUPPLY	TAPE BACKUP SYSTEM
ASPIRATOR	CRYOSTAT	GAS CHROMATOGRAPH	MOD, AIRWAY PRESS MON	POWER SUPPLY, CAMERA	TATTOO, ELECTRIC
ASPIRATOR, ENDOSCOPIC	CRYOSURGICAL UNIT	HANDLE, OTO/OPHTH	MOD, CO/PRESSURE	POWER SUPPLY, DRILL	TELEMETRY PROCESSOR
ASPIRATOR, LIPO	CYSTO-FLUORO	HANDPIECE, OPHTH	MOD, CO2/O2	POWER SUPPLY, LP10	TELEMETRY RECEIVER
ASPIRATOR, OPHTHAL	CYTOMETER	HANDPIECE, SHAVER	MOD, EKG	POWER SUPPLY/BED	TELEMETRY TRANSMITER
ASPIRATOR, ULTRASONIC	DEBRIDER	HEADLIGHT	MOD, EKG/RESP	POWERFILE	TENT, PED, AEROSOL
ASPIRATOR, UTERINE	DEFIB INTERFACE	HEART LUNG BYPASS UT	MOD, HEMODYNAMICS	PRESSURE/DOPPLER SYS	THERMOMETER
AUDIOMETER	DEFIB PADDLE ADAPTER	HEAT GUN	MOD, HOUSING, REMOTE	PRINTER	THERMOMETER, IVAC
BALANCE TEST SYSTEM	DEFIB PADDLES, EXT	HEAT SEAL	MOD, NIBP	PRINTER, LASER	THERMOMETER, TYMPANIC
BAR CODE READER	DEFIB PADDLES, INT	HEATER, IMMERSION	MOD, NIBP, ANES	PRINTER, VIDEO COLOR	THROMBECTOMY SYSTEM
BASSINET	DEFIB PROGRAMMER	HEATER, WAX	MOD, NIBP/SPO2	PRINTER, VIDEO MONO	THYROID UPTAKE SYS
BATCH BICARB SYSTEM	DEFIB, MON	HEATING PAD, WATER	MOD, OXIMETER, PULSE	PROJECTION POINTER	TIMER, COAGULATOR
BATH, PARAFFIN	DEFIB/MON	HEMATOCRIT READER	MOD, OXYGEN MONITOR	PROJECTOR, CHART, EYE	TIMER, PHOTOTHERAPY
BATH, THERMAL SPLINT	DEFIB/MON/PACE	HEMODIALYSIS UNIT	MOD, PHYSIOLOGIC	PULM FUNC ANALYZER	TOMOGRAPHY SYSTEM
BATH, WATER	DEFIBRILLATOR	HUMIDIFIER	MOD, PRESS/TEMP	PUMP PROGRAMMER	TOURNIQUET, REGULATED
BATH, WHIRL	DENSITOMETER	HYDROCOLLATOR	MOD, PRESSURE	PUMP, BREAST	TRACE GAS ANALYSIS
BATTERY CHARGER	DENT, US TOOTH CLEAN	HYPERTHERMIA, AIR	MOD, RECORDER	PUMP, ENDO	TRACTION UT, POWERED
BATTERY SUPPORT SYSM	DENT, VAC ADAPT	HYPERTHERMIA, WATER	MOD, SVO2	PUMP, ENTERAL FEEDING	TRANSDUCER, PRESSURE
BATTERY, LP10, PM	DENTAL AMALGAMATOR	HYPO/HYPERTHERMIA	MOD, VOLUME MON	PUMP, IA BALLOON	TRANSDUCER, TOCO
BED, BIRTHING	DENTAL ENGINE	HYPOTHERMIA CONTROL	MODEM, EKG	PUMP, SYRINGE	TREADMILL
BED, ELECTRIC	DENTAL HEATER	IMAGE CAPTURE SYSTEM	MON, CENT STA FILTER	PUMP, SYRINGE 360	UPS
BED, FLOTATION	DENTAL IMPLANT	IMAGE INTENSIFIER	MON, DEFIB	RADIOG SYS, CHEST	URINOMETER
BELLOWS, VENT	DENTAL SCANNER	IMAGE PROCESSOR	MONITOR, 3 CHAN, EXER	RADIOGRAPHIC SYSTEM	UROFLOWMETER
BILI-PHOTOMETER, UV	DENTAL TRIMMER	IMAGER, IR	MONITOR, CENTRAL STA	RADIOMETER	US BONE DENSITY
BIPAP	DENTAL X-RAY	IMPEDANCE METER	MONITOR, ECG	RECORDER, CHART	US CLEANER
BLENDER	DERMATOME	IMPRINTER	MONITOR, FETAL	RECORDER, CHART 2-CHN	US ENDOSCOPE
BLOOD FLOW DET, US	DIATHERMY, OPHTHALMIC	IMPRINTER, NUR	MONITOR, ICP	RECORDER, CHART 4-CHN	US IMAGER
BLOWER, CANOPY	DIATHERMY, US	INCU CONTROL	MONITOR, NERVE INTEGR	RECORDER, HOLTER	US PULSE UNIT
C.A.T. SYSTEM	DIELECTRIC SEALER	INCU DECK	MONITOR, NEUROLOGICAL	RECORDER, MULTICHANEL	US SURGICAL UNIT
CABINET, TREATMENT	DISPENSER, EMBEDDING	INCU STAND	MONITOR, NIBP	RECORDER, TAPE	US TRANSDUCER
CAMERA CONTROL	DISPENSER, DRUG	INCU WARMER HOOD	MONITOR, NIBP/SPO2	REFRACTOMETER	UV EXAMINING LIGHT
CAMERA FLASHER, ID	DISPENSER, FLUID	INCUBATOR, PLATELET	MONITOR, PC	REFRACTOMETER STAND	VACUUM ASSIST CLOSE
CAMERA, BABY, PORTRAIT	DRILL, BONE	INCUBATOR, LAB	MONITOR, PHYSIO, PORT	REFRIGERATOR	VACUUM DELIV SYS
CAMERA, FUNDUS	DRILL, MASTOID	INCUBATOR, TEST TUBE	MONITOR, PHYSIOLOGIC	REGULATOR, VACUUM	VACUUM REGULATOR
CAMERA, OPHTHALMIC	DRILL, SURGICAL	INCUBATOR, TRANSPORT	MONITOR, REMOTE CONTROL, RX	REMOTE CONTROL, ANES	VACUUM SOLUTION
CAMERA, VIDEO	DRIVE, DISK, LASER	INFANT WARMER	MONITOR/MAINFRAME	REMOTE CONTROL, TX	VENTILATION MONITOR
CAMERA, VIDEO IMAGE	DYNAMOMETER	INFLATOR, MATTRESS	MOTILITY MEAS SYS	REMOTE RF SYSTEM	VENTILATOR
CAPNOGRAPH	ECT	INFUSION PUMP	MOTION BASSINET	RF SYSTEM	VENTILATOR, ANES
CAPNOGRAPH, ANES	EEG ACQUISITION MOD	INFUSION PUMP, NXT	MOTOR, SAW	RF SYSTEM, DIGITAL	VENTILATOR, INFANT
CARDIAC COMPRESSOR	EEG COMPUTER	INFUSION PUMP, PCA	MRI SYSTEM	SCALE, ANALYTICAL	VIBRATOR, MASSAGE
CARDIAC MAPPING SYS	EEG, EMG COMPUTER	INJECTOR, CONTRAST	MULTIMETER, DIGITAL	SCALE, BODY FAT	VIDEO AMPLIFIER
CARDIAC OUTPUT TD	EKG APPLICATOR	INSUFFLATOR, CO2	NASOPHARYNGOSCOPE	SCALE, BED	VIDEO CAMERA CONTROL
CARDIAC OUTPUT/OXIMR	EKG, 3 CHAN	INTERCOM	NEBULIZER	SCALE, CHAIR	VIDEO MULTIPLEXER
C-ARM, PORTABLE	EKG, SINGLE CHANNEL	IRRADIATOR, BLOOD	NEBULIZER, ULTRASONIC	SCALE, DIAPER	VIDEO PROCESSOR
CART, MOBILE, ISO	ELEC HAIR CLIPPER	IRRIGATOR	NETWORK	SCALE, INFANT	VISION TESTER
CASSETTE PLAYER	ELECTRODIAGNOSTIC SY	ISOLATION CHAMBER	NITROGEN GAS METER	SCALE, SLING	VISUAL PULSE ANALYZER
CAST CUTTER VAC	ELECTROPHORESIS	ISOLATION TRANSFORMR	NUCLEOTOME	SCALE, SPECIMEN	VOLUME MONITOR
CAST CUTTER, ELECTRIC	EMBOSSER, CARD	KERATOMETER	NURSE CALL SYSTEM	SCALE, STANDING	WARMER, BLOOD
CATARACT EXTRACT UT	EMG	LARYNX, ARTIFICIAL	OCULOPLETHYSMOGRAPH	SCALE, STANDING, DIGIT	WARMER, CABINET
CELL SEPARATOR	EMG ACQUISITION MOD	LASER SMOKE EVAC	OPHTHAL SURG SYST	SCALE/SHAKER, BLOOD	WARMER, GEL
CELL WASHER	ENDOCOAGULATOR	LASER, ARG	OPHTHAL, INDIRECT	SCAVENGER, ANES	WARMER, INSTRUMENT
CENTRIFUGE	ENDOMETRIAL ABL SYS	LASER, CO2	OPHTHALMIC STAND	SEALER, THERMAL	WARMER, SOLUTION
CHAIR, DENTAL	ENDOSCOPE	LASER, DIODE	OPTICAL MODULE	SECURITY ACCESS SYS	WASHER, INSTRUMENT
CHAIR, EXAMINATION	EQUIPMENT CABINET	LASER, HELIUM-NEON	OSCILLOSCOPE MONITOR	SENSOR, CO2	WATER PURIF SYS

Joint Commission Statement

Briefings on Accreditation and Quality, July 1, 2017.

George Mills, MBA, FASHE, CEM, CHFM, CHSP, Joint Commission director of engineering at the time this policy was created – quoted here from a webinar, verbatim.

Q: With the changes to the standards, will equipment that's not found or is in use count in favor of or against completion percentage?

Mills: We've always said that if you go to a unit to do the work on equipment for service maintenance and it's on a patient and in use, we've never ever advocated taking it off a patient to see if it's working OK. But [say] you're there on time, on the date you're supposed to be doing the work, when the device is in use. At that point, we'd expect that you have some sort of policy to guide you as far as what the next steps are.

Steve [Grimes] gave some good examples of what those next steps could be as far as letting nursing know that as soon as this patient no longer needs this device, to call somebody at your shop so they can send somebody up to do the work.

But [since] you were there on time, you're going to get 100% credit for that. So you wouldn't consider yourself to be late servicing that equipment. In a similar situation (with equipment not found), you're in the unit the equipment is supposed to be in. You look for it and can't find it. Again, being driven by a strong policy, you go to nursing and say, "I'm looking for X device." They say, "Jeez, I haven't seen this up here in a long time." At that point, you put out an alert saying that you're looking for it.

And you have maybe a three step process where your first step was that you were on time, so you're taking the 100% as far as your recordkeeping goes. Maybe your policy says that within five days you return to the unit and look for it again and post it in the nurses' communications strategies asking nursing to help you find it. Maybe the third step is that you still can't find it, so you flag it as "deferred until found" or somehow indicate that it didn't receive its preventive maintenance (PM) because it couldn't be found. Ask nursing again to help you find it.

The key is that you are going to be taking 100% on your "on time" because you were on time, and you knew what it was. And the fact that you couldn't complete it wasn't your fault or a penalty to your shop. The key then becomes whether your policy is robust enough to still make sure that you capture that equipment when it does show up. If it doesn't show up after a second cycle, do you then remove it from your inventory as "not being in the building?" Maybe it went out with a patient to a nursing home or something like that; you never know.

The point is that for your 100% compliance calculations, if you were there to do the work on time, take the credit for being there on time. Your policy steps in and gives you the next steps, gives you the evidence of what to do next, because you couldn't service your equipment.

So a surveyor would be looking at your history and would say, "I see you are at 100%, but I see three things that were deferred because they were in use. What does your policy say?" Then if you can explain your policy back to the surveyor, everything should be fine because everything should be reconciled and driven by a written policy to get to that point.

****

Below is the last response I received from a recent attempt to address this issue with The Joint Commission.

"Dear Alan- I have spoken with everyone you reached out to and I am responding on behalf of those staff. We want to thank you for your efforts expended in your letter from January 24, 2018. It appears that you have thoroughly researched the topic of equipment maintenance rates. However, the Center for Medicare and Medicaid Services (CMS) has approved our maintenance rate of 100%. The Health care Organization has the responsibility to prove to the Joint Commission surveyor that they are meeting that 100% requirement. Regards, Dawn Glossa, Director Corporate Communications"

Contact the Joint Commission.
DGlossa@jointcommission.org, 630-792-5630
Gail Weinberger, Director, Accreditation and Certification, gweinberger@jointcommission.org, 630-792-5766
Anne Bauer, Field Director, Hospital Accreditation, abauer@jointcommission.org, 630-792-5863
Sharon Sprenger, Health care Quality Evaluation,

ssprenger@jointcommission.org, 630-792-5968

Mark R. Chassin, M.D., M.P.P., M.P.H., President, mchassin@jointcommission.org, 630-792-5650

Devil's Advocate

What the Joint Commission will tell you:

This Joint compliance standard is robust: it includes internal reporting requirements and follow up.

This standard has been approved by the CMS.

Equipment not located for inspections must be reported to affected departments and include follow up to assure completion of periodic maintenance inspections.

This policy rewards departments for their efforts in complying, recognizing that different institutions present a range of obstacles that are typically found in healthcare.

The surveyor always has the authority to drill down and follow wherever the evidence leads.

However, survey organizations, including The Joint, will not explain or acknowledge the following.

Focusing compliance on adherence to a schedule, rather than numbers of devices actually inspected on time, enables care facilities to budget maintenance departments ("Biomed") more stress-free: reporting real numbers can make an administration look bad, lending support to an increase in funding for maintenance – not a position administrations want to be in. This is one reason hospitals prefer a standard that enables an easier 100% compliance. And a Biomed administrator can more easily demand that their staff meet a schedule than they can demand technicians increase the number of devices inspected in an hour.

I can fully appreciate how difficult it is to challenge The Joint: in some cases, your job may even be at stake. I understand, I've been there.

A History of This Subject

This is an early (2004) response from The Joint to my proposal for calculating maintenance compliance.

Last is their current response: much more evasive.

```
From: <JFishbeck@jcaho.org>
```

```
To: "Concerned Connections"
<info@concernedconnections.org>
Cc: <BBerek@jcaho.org>;
<rawise@jcaho.org>; <jloeb@jcaho.org>
```

Sent: Thursday, January 08, 2004 7:47 PM

Subject: Submission – Medical Equipment Management

Though your rational was most eloquently presented, it was felt that since the healthcare organizations we accredit vary widely in size, complexity, operations, and risk, our standards rarely are able to prescribe one particular method of compliance of the type presented in your letter. In addition it was felt that prescribing one method of compliance could limit development of other ideas.

Each setting we accredit may have different operational variables and are expected to customize their medical equipment management programs to optimize their effectiveness. The definitions for "compliance" provided your letter appear to be relevant to your setting; as always our on-site process would confirm if they are indeed effective.

Finally, it was felt the concepts and definitions you presented may be useful as examples to others, and perhaps you should explore providing input to groups that develop guidance and management strategy documents for similar settings (i.e. large hospitals, in this case). Some suggestions would be ASHE 's "Maintenance Management for Medical Equipment", the AAMI publication "EQ-56" or the AAMI publication "Joint Commission Standards for Clinical Engineering Departments" by Bob Stieffel. These would be appropriate venues for this type of information.

Sincerely,
John Fishbeck
Associate Director
Division of Standards and Survey Methods

***

It's Not a Fun Subject

The following is The Joint's response.
from: Glossa, Dawn <DGlossa@jointcommission.org>
to: Alan Pakaln <alanpakaln@gmail.com>
cc: "Glossa, Dawn" <DGlossa@jointcommission.org>
date: Feb 9, 2018, 3:19 PM
subject: RE: External E-Mail: Re: Joint Maintenance Article
mailed-by: jointcommission.org
signed-by: jointcommission.onmicrosoft.com
Dear Alan-

Thank you for clarifying your intentions. I have spoken with everyone you reached out to and I am responding on behalf of those staff.

We want to thank you for your efforts expended in your letter from January 24, 2018. It appears that you have thoroughly researched the topic of equipment maintenance rates.

However, the Center for Medicare and Medicaid Services (CMS) has approved our maintenance rate of 100%. The Healthcare Organization has the responsibility to prove to the Joint Commission surveyor that they are meeting that 100% requirement.

Regards,
Dawn
Dawn Glossa, MPA
Director Corporate Communications
Certified Change Agent
The Joint Commission

BMET and Clinical Engineer

Over a one year period beginning in 2018, I mailed – sometimes posted, others emailed - journalists plus about 800 administrators who oversee hospital safety. I received only a few – all positive – responses.

It's Not a Fun Subject

```
The letter I wrote
```

BMET and Clinical Engineer

Joint Commission Accreditation

I am a biomedical engineer, concerned about The Joint Commission's oversight of medical equipment maintenance. I have 30+ years experience overseeing the application of medical technology in New York City hospitals (Bellevue, St. Luke's-Roosevelt-Mt. Sinai). I have participated in many accreditation surveys, and have written about this issue, both in journals and to The Joint Commission. See their response:

https://jointcommissionaccreditation.org/

Patients are at increased risk because, when medical equipment inspection rates are not tracked, equipment is not inspected on time and failures may increase. Of the 21,000 Joint Commission surveyed institutions, no one knows the inspection rate for medical equipment – not despite Joint standards, but because of them. Because there is no available inspection data, no one knows how this plays out in terms of reported incidents: incidents must be reported, but maintenance completion rates are not required.

How is this possible?

The policy:
The Joint Commission accreditation standard for medical equipment periodic maintenance is 100%. However, The Joint does not require 100% of the equipment to be inspected on time; their policy requires that maintenance technicians follow an inspection schedule 100% of the time. A technician can adhere to a schedule regardless of the number of equipment pieces that are inspected: miss some equipment in a scheduled location, you can just move on to the next scheduled location. Technicians are motivated to stay on schedule to avoid being cited on a survey.

Inspecting 100% of the medical equipment on time is not just difficult for many institutions, it is virtually impossible to achieve because some equipment invariably is "missing" during inspections: "floaters" like IV pumps travel from one department to another, equipment may be stolen or transferred to another department, rentals are returned, staff may hide equipment because of perceived shortages, a department may send something out for repair, equipment can be in use on a patient, or perhaps maintenance technicians are just not as thorough as they might be.

The problem:
Equipment not inspected can be "missing" or just not looked for during the prescribed inspection period. These numbers do not become part of the compliance calculation and reporting, even though some of the uninspected equipment may be in use on patients.

Why would The Joint set a standard of 100%, when it is virtually impossible to inspect all equipment 100% on time? Two reasons.
1. 100% means The Joint does not need to justify setting anything lower (95%?; why not 96%? Or 94%?). What science could they use in their rationale?
2. The Joint can have just one standard for everyone: smaller facilities (with lower numbers of "missing" equipment), and larger facilities (with higher numbers of "missing" equipment).

The reason this standard is bad.
No one can tell from compliance reporting what the actual level of equipment inspections is, nor can anyone see how long some equipment remains uninspected. Also, less meaningful data means less diligence: what incentive to improve is there when there is an approved, guaranteed, and easy way to achieve 100%?

Reasonable alternatives?
First, show real numbers so everyone can know what the actual rate of inspected equipment is. If the rate is 95%, state that, and state why it is 95% and not higher. Second, show the percent and breakdown of equipment not located. If the inspection rate is 95%, explain the 5% so that everyone can assess the quality of inventory, and more clearly track and focus on what is not inspected and why it isn't.

Periodic compliance reporting should look something like this. Using a total inventory quantity of 1,000 with 95% of inventory inspected on time, the remaining 5%, or 50 pieces, are past due. This uninspected or unlocated equipment (insufficient staffing is included here) should be explained – e.g., in shop, on patient, or other - along with numbers of intervals missed. And of course, at some point, equipment that is not located for some prescribed period can - after findings are reported, reviewed and signed off by various personnel - be removed from inventory.

What policy can The Joint Commission establish to promote maintenance safety, and be appropriate to all? If The Joint had been collecting real data for a period of time, perhaps a meaningful percent could now be set as a standard, tailored for different institution types and sizes. But as things stand now, meeting a standard must mean you meet or better the institution's benchmark: e.g. 95% compliant with 5% uninspected or missing, means that the institution must meet or better those numbers in the next survey. Or satisfactorily explain why it can't.

Real maintenance compliance numbers, trended over time, will place a clearer focus on the efforts made to improve performance. Real numbers measure actual results, and the surveyor always has the prerogative of accepting explanations for numbers that deviate from the norm.

The proposed fix keeps the issue of unlocated inventory front and center where it should be. What incentive is there to improve if – as is the case now – you rely on a system that all but guarantees 100%? When it's likely you are not.

What you don't know can hurt. I encourage you to look into this and ask The Joint Commission for their rationale. To contact me - home landline is: . (Note, I don't usually pick up if I don't recognize the number – too much phone-spam; so please leave a message and I will call back).
https://jointcommissionaccreditation.org/
Thank you, Alan Pakaln

Organizations contacted

In 2018 and 2019, I contacted approximately 900 individuals – MDs, hospital safety officers, journalists – in an attempt to incite some interest in how maintenance compliance was and still is, calculated.

BMET and Clinical Engineer

24x7 Magazine	Duke University Hospital
Agency for Healthcare Research and Quality (AHRQ)	ECRI
AHME New	Emergency Consultants PSO, LLC
Akron Children's Hospital	Encompass Health Patient Safety Organization
AMA Medical Student Section	Encore
American Medical Foundation Patient Safety	FDA
American Society for Health Care Risk Management (ASHRM)	Florida Academic Healthcare Patient Safety
Anesthesia Patient Safety Foundation	Forbes
Answers Media Network	Garden State Patient Safety Center
ASA	George Washington Medical Faculty Associates
Ascension Healthcare Patient Safety	Health Catalyst, Inc
Association for the Advancement of Medical Instrumentation (AAMI)	Health Watch USAsm
Association of Health Care Journalists	Healthcare Council of Western Pennsylvania
Atlanta VAMC	Healthcare Systems Engineering Institute
Aunt Minnie. Com	HealthcareScene.com & HITMC.com
AVAHCS	HealthTech Magazine
Barnes-Jewish Hospital	Hospital for Special Surgery
Bassett Medical Center	Hospital Quality Institute
Baylor College of Medicine	HPM Department
Becker's Hospital Review	Illinois Department of Public Health
Boston Children's Hospital	Illinois Health and Hospital Association
Boston Globe	InquisitHealth
Brigham and Women's Hospital	Institute for Healthcare Improvement
Brooklyn Hospital Center	Institute for Innovation in Health
California Arthritis Partnership Program	Institute for Patient Safety
California Hospital Association	Institute for Safe Medication Practices
Cancer Treatment Centers of America	Institute for Safe Medication Practices
Catholic Health Services of Long Island	Institute for Safe Medication Practices (ISMP)
Cedars-Sinai	Intermountain Healthcare
Center for Evidence and Practice Improvement	Internet Health Management
Center for Patient Safety	Investigative Reporters and Editors
Center for Quality Improvement and Patient Safety (CQuIPS)	Jefferson Hospital
Centers for Medicare and Medicaid Services	Johns Hopkins All Children's Hospital
Centralized Hospital Intake Program	Johns Hopkins Bloomberg School of Public Health
Chicago Sun-Times	Johns Hopkins Hospital
Chicago Tribune	Joint Commission Journal
Child Health Patient Safety Organization	Kaiser Permanente Research
Children's Hospital Colorado	Kaiser Permanente School of Medicine
Children's Hospital of Pittsburgh of UPMC	LA County Department of Health
Cleveland Clinic	LA Times
Cleveland Clinic, Medicine Institute	Laurabell.com
Cleveland Clinic, Quality & Patient Safety Institute	Los Angeles Biomedical Research Institute
Colorado Department of Healthcare Policy	Maimonides Medical Center
Community Health Center, Inc./ReachMD	Massachusetts Department of Public Health
Consumers Union	Massachusetts General Hospital
Consumers Union Safe Patient Project Network	Mathematica Policy Research
DARTNet Institute	Mayo Clinic Health System
Data Across Sectors for Health	Medical School College of Engineering University of Michigan
Delaware Division of Public Health	Medicare
Department of Health and Mental Hygiene	MedStar Health
Duke University Health System	MedStar Health

It's Not a Fun Subject

MHA Health Foundation	Robert Wood Johnson Foundation
MHA Keystone Center	Robert Wood Johnson University Hospital
Michigan Department of Community Health	Rush University College of Nursing
Michigan Health Information Network Shared Services	San Diego Health Connect
Mid-Atlantic Patient Safety	Seattle Times
Modern Healthcare	SF Chronicle
Montefiore Hudson Valley	Society of Corporate Compliance and Ethics
Mothers Against Medical Error	Society!for!Simulation!in!Healthcare
Mount Sinai	St. Francis Hospital
Nassau University Medical Center	Stanford Health Care
National Committee for Quality Assurance	Stanford University
National Institutes of Health	Stanford University Department of Medicine
Nebraska Hospital Association	Stanford University School of Medicine
New England Quality Care Alliance	STONY BROOK UNIVERSITY HOSPITAL
New Jersey Department of Health	Strategic Radiology Patient Safety
New York Times	Surgical Outcomes & Quality Improvement Center
New York University	Tennessee Center for Patient Safety
Newsday	Texas Hospital Association
New York-Presbyterian	The Baltimore Sun
NORTH SHORE UNIVERSITY HOSPITAL	THE BROOKLYN HOSPITAL CENTER
NorthShore	The Detroit Free Press
Northwell Health	The James M. Anderson Center for Health Systems Excellence
Northwestern Medical Group	The Joint Commission
Northwestern University	The Leapfrog Group
Nursing Alliance for Quality Care	The National Quality Forum
NY Post	Today's Practice Magazine
NY State Dept Health	UCLA
NY Times	UCSF
NYC HEALTH + HOSPITALS	University Hospital
NYT	University of Chicago Medicine
NYU Langone	University of Iowa
NYU Lutheran Medical Center	University of Michigan Health System
Ohio Department of Health	University of Michigan Hospitals
Ohio Patient Safety Institute	University of Pennsylvania
Ohio State University Wexner Medical Center	University of Pittsburgh Medical Center
Oregon Public Health Department	UPMC Presbyterian Shadyside, Pittsburgh
Partners HealthCare	USA Today
Patient Safety Action Network	USC ANNENBERG
Patient Safety Movement Foundation	Vanderbilt University Medical Center
Penn State Health	Veterans Administration
Pennsylvania Department of Health	Virginia Hospital and Healthcare Association
Pennsylvania Patient Safety Authority	Wall Street Journal
Permanente Medical Group	Wall Street Raw Radio
PHELPS MEMORIAL HOSPITAL CENTER	Washington Advocates for Patient Safety
Philadelphia Enquirer	Washington Post
Politico	Washington State Department of Health
Press Ganey	Weill Cornell Medical College
Project HOPE	WellStar Health System
Public Health Reaching Across Sectors	Westchester Medical Center
Quality Center Patient Safety	WHITE PLAINS HOSPITAL
Quality Circle for Healthcare	Xtelligent Media

BMET and Clinical Engineer

Addendum
Journal Article One

The following is a journal article I wrote, published by AAMI, Association for the Advancement of Medical Instrumentation in 2004. Among other things, it briefly describes the associated method of risk assessment.

The Three Critical Issues I've Learned in 23 Years in Clinical Engineering

My career in Clinical Engineering began in 1979, at Bellevue Hospital, a municipal facility of New York City. I chose Bellevue for the broad experience I was sure I would receive, the most impressive of which was witnessing technology's march into medicine. I went on to other institutions, and over time, concluded that equipment maintenance was the most problematic area of responsibility I faced. And of maintenance, the least favorite tasks I performed were risk assessments, and compliance calculation.

There were good reasons for this unpopularity: I found risk assessment to be subjective, even arbitrary, and achieving compliance was at best difficult, and at worst a game of hide and seek. Added to these problems, I often found little administrative support, or appreciation for the issues that were growing more complex every year. Today's medical technology oversight includes standards, but few clear paths to follow when it comes to implementing those standards. The following are three issues I have found to be most critical, and my suggestions for addressing them.

I. Risk Assessment

Ignorance may be bliss, but effective assessments cannot be made if the assessment methodology is a contrivance designed for ease of use. Methodologies must be standardized: factoring in the various subjective decisions that must be made so we can clearly see the effect those decisions have on the conclusions we make.

One formula I have found in use, $E + C + (M + F + U)/3$, relies on the following weighted equipment variables: function (E), application (C), maintenance requirement (M), likelihood of failure (F), and environment (U). Plug in the numbers, and out comes the conclusion. But each of these variables calls for an educated guess, and three of them (M, F, and U), are weighted equally in the formula. Formula-based methodologies and applications relying on pattern recognition or forms of artificial intelligence (neural nets, fuzzy logic, etc.), have been used to address variables inherent in the maintenance of medical equipment. While a formula may be used only as a guide, it may not be. And though it may take into account significant issues, it represents an opinion that you may not feel free to alter.

You cannot, with absolute certainty, determine a device's "critical nature," what the "consequence of failure" will be, or what effect location will have on a patient's treatment, without including subjective analysis. Analysis that includes subjective observation is often necessary, but offering that analysis as absolute is misleading, and can distract the reviewer from thinking about the significant factors comprising the assessment. Subjective assessments demand a visible process.

Today, we may remove from a maintenance program certain devices, based not on risk assessment per se, but on other rationales. Advanced technologies and manufacturing capabilities have improved to the extent that we may not regularly inspect every pressure transducer, catheter, temperature probe, or other disposables, attachments, and ancillary devices. These pieces are often essential to the clinical integrity of a procedure, yet in some cases, we make a decision not to manage them the way we do other pieces of equipment. Risk assessment can take into account many variables including reliability, production run problems, past history, manufacturer's recommendations, calibration, lubrication, part replacement, consequence of failure, how apparent a failure is, built-in self test, equipment age, physical environment, user technique and experience. We can establish the criteria. The issue is how to use them without overwhelming the user, and without hiding the facts.

The following four variable groups are presented here as critical in directing risk assessment.

1. 100% self testing. Check with manufacturers, but a 100% electronic device that performs a self-test on startup is often sufficient to assure operational integrity.

2. Failure apparent to the user. A problem that is not apparent to the user can stay hidden until a maintenance inspection is performed. Sometimes this characteristic is obvious (compare the verification procedure for insufflator inflation pressure to that for

oto/ophthalmoscope quality of light), and sometimes it is not, but this critical issue demands resolution.

3. Calibration, lubrication, and parts replacement. If it's required, it's scheduled.

4. Consequence of failure to the patient. In some cases this is clear, as an insufflator compared with an oto/ophthalmoscope (great, and slight), in others it is not as clear, as in a transport cardiac monitor, or EKG machine.

Table 1 demonstrates maintenance requirements ascertained for four sample devices. Working out the various permutations will result in a finite number which can be used as a reference either on paper, or in a database expression. Remember, this format is not a formula. It is, in a sense, a triage guide, weeding out those devices whose maintenance characteristics are most readily defined. Its structure provides definition and flexibility, and it forces the user to become involved.

II. Maintenance Compliance Calculation

Utilizing a formula methodology for risk assessment, but not for inventory management, is like locking the door after the horse has left the barn. The term "inventory" must be defined in absolute terms to effectively track compliance, or to make quality comparisons between institutions.

Theoretically, "compliance" is a ratio of the number of devices that are inspected on time, divided by the total number of devices in the maintenance program—this is easy math. I say theoretically though, because we have not defined what "total number" stands for—this is the tricky part. In the real world, the denominator in compliance calculations is defined by each user. The "total number" could stand for all devices in the maintenance program, or all devices that have been located within a certain time period. In other words, nothing prevents a department from discounting all devices not located during a one month inspection sweep. Here is the issue—percent compliance can be increased without increasing the number of maintenance inspections: report "compliance" as a percent of devices in your maintenance program with inspections completed "as scheduled."

BMET and Clinical Engineer

100% Self Test	Failure Apparent	Maintenance Required (calibration, lubrication, parts replacement)	Consequence of Failure (direct, and indirect-critical environment, likelihood of causing confusion during critical procedure)	Maintenance Determination
YES	APPARENT	NO	LITTLE	Maintenance Not Required
N/A	N/A	YES	N/A	Maintenance Required *
NO	NOT APPARENT	NO	GREAT	Short Maintenance Interval **
NO	APPARENT	NO	MODERATE	Resolve ***

Table 1 *demonstrates maintenance requirements ascertained for four sample devices.*
* Interval depends on maintenance required by the manufacturer.
** Establishing exact intervals is not the issue here.
*** The fact that a failure would be apparent to the user, and regular maintenance is not required, does not permit an accurate determination because Consequence of Failure is MODERATE. Miscellaneous variables such as repair history, equipment age, physical environment, and diagnostic use must be considered.

Let's say it's November 2003, and you print out a list of 100 devices, which have inspections due that month. Like a good manager, you assign these to your technicians, and like good technicians, they perform their work and enter their work orders. Now it is December 1, and you run your compliance report and find that of the 100 devices handed out, 95 were inspected. You report 95% maintenance compliance for that month, and go on to the next month. So far, so good. For this example, let us assume that all of the devices in your program have a one year inspection interval. One year later, November 2004, you ask for everything that is due in the current month. This time only 95, of the original 100 devices, are handed out to the technicians.

The five not completed from a year ago (lost, stolen, returned to a vendor, hidden, or not having sufficient staff to locate) do not come up—this month or in any other month—because you only ask for devices that have due dates for the current month and the current year. In other words, each and every month, devices "not located" are effectively removed from the maintenance program and from compliance calculations. Relying on this method continually adjusts the work you have to do, to the work you are able to do. Performing calculations in this manner will increase compliance, not by virtue of having inspected more devices, but by reducing on paper, the devices in use.

There are no established standards for how you must treat the denominator in compliance calculations—you could include all devices (generating an unrealistically low number), or exclude all not

Addendum

located each month, as in the example previously mentioned (not a true reflection of maintenance in your facility). These are the extremes. There is a middle ground.

Draw a line representing the oldest due date—to the most future due date, and designate a period (18 months for example), removing from calculation (not from inventory) devices that have not been located for that period (Table 2). The time period should be long enough to reasonably allow equipment to be found. Note: "# of Devices," the area below the curve, represent devices included in the periodic maintenance program.

The critical issues are: to define the cut-off point, report devices removed from compliance calculation (as a percent of inventory), and report that number to the Environment of Care Committee as you would compliance. The report would look something like: 95% compliant, 4.5% devices not located. The point is, if the numbers reported were 95% compliant, 35% of inventory not located, a red flag should go up somewhere.

Equipment not accounted for can be lost, stolen, returned to a vendor, errors in inventory, hidden, or simply the result of not having enough resources to do the job. Some of this is "forgivable," and some of it is not. Not standardizing this procedure skews data—there is no distinction between devices that truly do not exist, and those simply not found. Without making this distinction, you cannot effectively track performance, the Joint Commission (JCAHO) cannot accurately compare one institution to another, and patients may be placed at increased risk.

III. Administrative Oversight

"Good people are where you find them," but don't leave the selection of technology oversight to good looks and politics. If your key technology person is reporting to the same administrator who oversees laundry, security, and housekeeping, with all due respect, that may be the wrong person. Thirty years ago, medical technology was less prevalent and less complex. If a power plug failed, the maintenance person who fixed the lights and kept the boiler going, repaired it. Other failures were referred to the manufacturer. This starting point has a remnant carried forward to today's high-tech environment. In some institutions, administrators overseeing food service, security, laundry, patient transport, housekeeping, and the maintenance department, also oversee the environment of medical technology. These administrators may have neither the expertise, nor the interest, to look beyond the quarterly summary reports they receive. The result of this inattention to detail can be increased risk to patients and increased costs to hospitals.

The excuse often used to explain this kind of failure within a bureaucratic system is: "It's not the individual's fault, it's the system." The failure of an institution may not be incompetence as much as a flawed table of organization. The Clinical Engineering department head (or vendor) should report to someone who understands patient care and the clinical environment—whether physician, PhD, or nursing director.

Addendum

Summary

Department directors are often caught between cost and service. Help them, not by increasing expenditures, but by building into the institution fabric definitions they can use. Make risk assessment something everyone can see and understand. Make compliance calculation show the whole picture including the integrity of your inventory. And place administrative oversight into the hands of those who best relate to it.

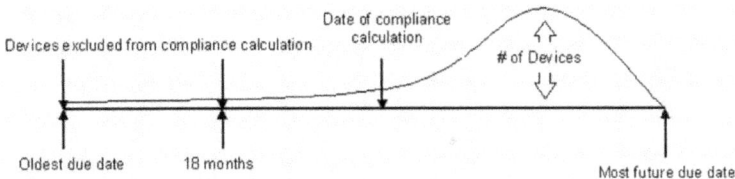

Table 2. A line representing the oldest due date to the most future due date, and designating a period.

BMET and Clinical Engineer

Addendum: Journal Article Two

Proposed: A Standard Clinical Engineering Review Procedure

(Biomedical Instrumentation & Technology 2006; 40:315–318).

Those overseeing clinical engineering (CE) functions at the top policy level—the Food and Drug Administration (FDA), the Joint Commission on Accreditation of Healthcare Organizations (JCAHO), and others in the profession—depend on sporadic assessments of nonstandard samplings of data when analyzing CE functions such as maintenance compliance, risk and failure analysis, and inventory management. This methodology results in the following: a fragmented view of operational functions, a limited view of the interrelationships of CE functions, and policies that reflect assumptions of equipment reliability.

The oversight of equipment maintenance, including the development of JCAHO standards, relies on data sampling, surveyor discretion, a range of policy reviews, and a presentation format that does not make apparent the interrelationships of CE functions or the status of internal policy reviews. In other words, the scope of CE services is monstrously large, interconnected, and involves large groups of people each with their own viewpoint and communication style. I propose that we address this situation by getting everyone and everything together on the same page, discussing and recording the results in a way that is clear and easy to share, and then circulating the document. This proposal is not easy to implement, but it addresses a wide range of shortcomings. Among them are the following:

1. Sporadic data sampling—This results in procedural reviews that are incomplete and not directly representative of service functions. What an equipment management plan states, and what is delivered can have two distinctly different outcomes.

Nobody really knows how risk assessments are performed in hospitals, or even how a critical piece of data like percent maintenance compliance is derived. It is currently possible for a hospital reporting a high maintenance compliance to have a greater percent of equipment requiring maintenance due for inspection than a hospital with a low percent or noncompliant status has (e.g. simply discount *all* equipment not located at the time of calculation).

Nobody knows the condition of hospital inventory and service records—what percentage of inventory cannot be located due to insufficient staff or mismanagement, or because it is not on the premises. Among other things, these data can have a direct impact on risk assessment, maintenance procedures, analysis of the effectiveness of maintenance, compliance calculation, failure analysis, the use of hazard alerts and recalls, and the length of time equipment can be expected to last, which in turn affects new technology planning and treatment costs.

Automated data retrieval via the Internet would increase data collection from health care organizations and would simplify many tasks, including accreditation surveys.

2. CE Functions—The separate functions that CE performs, such as risk assessment, maintenance, and equipment planning, are rarely analyzed in a way that makes inconsistencies in policy development obvious.

Reviewing CE functions and policies as separate issues and reporting the current state of development and future plans as individual phenomenon, does not allow for a comprehensive viewing of the interrelationships of CE functions. A standardized presentation that includes all major functions and policies would make issues more visible to more people. Such a presentation would also force a continual and more orderly review of all issues regardless of popularity.

3. Sporadic reporting—This restricts institutions in their ability to share significant data quickly and effectively with oversight groups and other institutions. Many types of issues, such as equipment failure and user errors, parts acquisition, and preventive maintenance corrective actions, are made available to other institutions on a voluntary basis only.

4. The monster in the closet—Balancing cost and patient safety. Under loose controls, cost consciousness can influence, subtly and insidiously, the way problem areas are interpreted, turning complex environments into "opportunities" for simplified administration of services (e.g. department mergers, department management downsizing, outsourcing) and cookie-cutter cost containment. There is real incentive and real ability to bypass effective issue assessment, instead of depending on surveys that rely on data sampling.

The problem is not the conversion of raw data into generalized assessments. Condensing and summarizing data for review purposes is a practical necessity in any oversight process involving large amounts of data and groups of people. At issue is the method used in collecting and displaying that data: determining the type and quantity of information necessary for meaningful oversight, and the form in which the information is presented. The FDA relies on voluntary failure reporting, "Medical Device Reporting" for manufacturers, importers, and user facilities and MEDWATCH for consumers and practitioners (Center for Devices and Radiological Health / CDRH, updated September 22, 2002). The JCAHO also relies on voluntary failure reporting, "Sentinel Events...involving death or serious physical or psychological injury, or the risk thereof."

Addressing the problems

You cannot clearly see the solutions if you cannot clearly see the problems.

Adopt a standardized review procedure to help ensure that everyone in the CE profession has access to a more complete representation of CE functions, to observe the interrelationships of CE functions, and to review more realistically the effectiveness and value of any one function. There are three basic areas that need to be addressed:

1. Base policy and (to some degree) accreditation on data that are collected on a continuous basis, rather than depending on periodic research and the intuition of inspection surveyors.

2. Assess the interrelationships of CE functions. Remember that functions such as inventory management, risk assessment, and maintenance compliance are linked one way or another to each other and to patient safety and resource expenditures.

3. Create a consistent presentation format. Because a standardized review of policies and standards necessarily would be broad in scope and would involve many people with different views, a standardized presentation format would help ensure that everyone is using the same language, referring to the same specific points, and addressing all the relevant issues.

A New Environment, Again

We have entered a new era where business and engineering advances have formed partnerships with hospitals. This is reflected in increased demand for and availability of new and costly technologies, strict reimbursement formulas, and increased reliability of technologies.

It is no secret that one challenge facing CE services has migrated from the adoption of new technologies to the adoption of improved design and manufacturing methodologies. We do not inspect each physiologic sensor prior to use. We do not periodically inspect all AC operated patient care devices. Trust in manufacturing, backed by historiography, enables us to "violate" what just years ago were pillars in ethics.

Increased reliability on technology, coupled with data sampling oversight, has contributed to an environment in which CE service providers assume greater authority over their procedural methodology and participate in an accreditation survey that is more craps game than survey. That is to say, CE administrators can influence outcomes by design and selection of operational initiatives, and surveyors pick and choose the trail they "dig down." This does not mean that CE receives no scrutiny or guidance, but the integrity and form of analysis and reporting are left mainly to those doing the maintenance and program design. A JCAHO mandate is to educate; however, the student has become the authority and the exam is left to chance.

Addendum: Journal Article Two

This is not good management design, but it is understandable how the system got this way. Consider the complexity of this environment—the matrix of efficacy, cost, and safety. Also, visualize it from the perspective of JCAHO: new and changing technologies; a mix of inside and outside service providers; large and small full-service and specialty patient care facilities; and a range of professional organizations, manufacturers, and service staff capabilities. Now administer effective risk assessment, maintenance protocols, and data collection and analysis— all in an atmosphere of live-or-die cost containment.

The JCAHO and the FDA certainly recognize that they cannot micromanage medical equipment servicing. As a result, they focus their attention on the bigger picture, hoping for trickle-down effects.

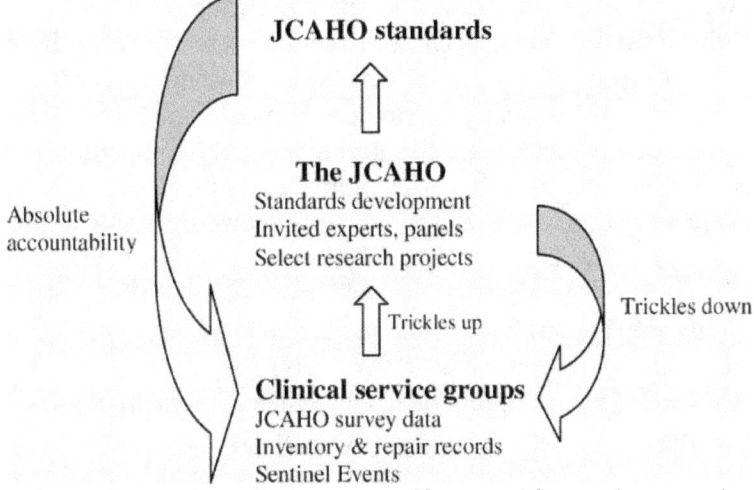

But there is a gap. Voluntary efforts aside, only samples of information travel from the operations level to those with the ultimate say-so. The result: A view at the top is sporadic and fractured. Trickle up data influence policy development and nobody really knows how much of what trickles down (see the Figure).

Everyone—CE service providers and the JCAHO—copes with complex and changing environments, and policies and standards that shift to accommodate change. It is a human environment with human reactions.

Four fears CE service providers have of standardizing procedures:

1. It will cost more money.

2. It may bring lower functioning service providers up in terms of quality, but may bring (my) higher functioning service down.

3. It will stifle my ability to address critical issues in ways that relate to my specific environment.

4. It will cost me precious time, reduce what little control I have over my department, and force me to pay attention to bureaucratic form rather than to the staff screaming at me for service.

Fears such as these are not easily addressed. One could, however, look to wisdom in an axiom such as: "A more controlled environment is a good one only if it truly offers greater control."

What controls are in place in the current environment of care? How the JCAHO oversees CE functions is determined by how the JCAHO controls its standards development—and vice versa. The information for this oversight process comes from a patchwork of thousands of hospitals, plus the input of JCAHO staff and invited experts in the field. From the viewpoint of this proposal, an effective review process can only be achieved if all involved parties can see and can understand all the issues. Without a holistic approach to oversight, "management by crisis" can dictate that the issue screaming the loudest will generate the greatest activity. That is as true for policy development as it is for service.

In order to interpret one CE function, all functions and relationships that make up the practice of clinical engineering must be clearly visible. You would not dismantle a sophisticated piece of technology without having the appropriate service manual. Why should our behavior be any different in overseeing the set of interdependent CE functions?

Addendum: Journal Article Two

	CE functions	Interrelationships									
		1	2	3	4	5	6	7	8	9	10
1	Inventory management					x	x		x	x	
2	Repair & failure analysis			x	x		x	x	x	x	x
3	Risk assessment analysis				x	x				x	x
4	Maintenance scheduling					x				x	x
5	Maintenance compliance calculation									x	
6	Recall, hazard, failure reporting				x				x	x	
7	Maintenance effectiveness analysis			x	x	x			x		x
8	Equipment life span analysis									x	x
9	Treatment efficacy (patient safety)			x	x				x		
10	Efficiency monitoring (cost containment)				x				x	x	

Table 1. *Clinical engineering (CE) functions and their interrelationships.*

Implementation

Implementation means creating definition; it does not mean "set in stone." When a system evolves, there must be mechanisms that permit core changes, as in naming CE service functions. Nothing remains the same. Standardizing nomenclature and a presentation format involves defining a structure that makes visible proposed alterations and includes the format used to track changes.

1. Make the viewing of CE functions and their interrelationships (Table 1), as in the following example, part of a formal review process.

Inventory management impacts maintenance compliance calculation, recall, hazard, failure reporting, and equipment life-span analysis—which, in turn, impact treatment efficacy (patient safety) and efficiency (cost containment).

Repair data impacts risk assessment, scheduled maintenance, recall, hazard, failure reporting, maintenance effectiveness analysis, and equipment lifespan analysis—which, in turn, impact treatment efficacy and efficiency.

Risk assessment impacts scheduled maintenance and maintenance compliance—which, in turn, impact treatment efficacy and efficiency.

2. Maintain a standard presentation format. The tenet underlying this proposal is that some functions, such as quality of inventory records and risk assessment, directly impact others, such as maintenance scheduling and compliance calculation. These functions affect treatment efficacy and cost. Also, there are more functions and issues than can be analyzed and discussed conveniently by groups of people with varying degrees of expertise and involvement—without a

standard recording and tracking format. The example shown in Table 2 is used only to illustrate the idea.

3. Develop an online system of data collection, so monitored issues are reported on an ongoing basis. Device nomenclature, data collection, and safety are just some of the issues involved in this stage of the implementation process.

4. Place the implemented changes on the Web and print, circulate, and discuss the issues highlighted by all involved parties.

Table 2. *Recording and tracking format for clinical engineering (CE) functions.*

CE Function	Interrelationships	Discussion	Results

Objectives in Adopting a Standard Clinical Engineering Review Procedure

1. To better view and understand the relationships of different clinical engineering (CE) functions and to emphasize the effects that changes to one have on others. Creating standards to manage the process of reviewing CE functions also will enable deficiencies in the reliability of these functions to be seen more easily.

2. To better resolve efficacy issues (e.g. risk assessment) that arise from purely economic issues (cost containment).

3. To better track the work by different groups (e.g. Joint Commission on Accreditation of

Healthcare Organizations, Association for the Advancement of Medical Instrumentation,

ECRI, and Food and Drug Administration) on multiple issues.

4. To better share information of various CE functions within the network of hospitals and oversight organizations, and to present this work in a form that encourages participation and promotes greater understanding.

Addendum: Journal Article Three

A Critical Factor

Out of necessity, hospitals must balance risk with expenditures. A reasonable and structured approach should be relied on when addressing scheduled maintenance costs.

The popular recommendation for Alternative Equipment Management (AEM) risk assessment calls for comparing two primary characteristics: *Likelihood of Failure*, and *Consequence of Failure*. I propose replacing *Likelihood of Failure* with *Failure Apparent to the Operator* for the following reasons. *Likelihood of Failure* - when clearly identified using service data - is relevant information that can be effective in prescribing maintenance, e.g. necessary battery replacement. However, *guessing* at *Likelihood of Failure* on an equipment component level is subjective and may not be as meaningful in directing maintenance. I propose that *appearance*, or *Failure Apparent to the Operator*, offers a clearer path to assessing actual risk.

I recognize that *Failure Apparent to the Operator* may not seem as clear or reasonable a risk criteria as *likelihood of failure*. However I believe that the observation of failure as it relates to risk can be more clearly established and that in practice it is a clearer indicator of risk - a paradigm shift in viewing.

Failure data from service records - *Likelihood of Failure* – can be very useful and should be applied as a separate indicator for maintenance rather than a risk criteria. A specific issue can indicate the need for individualized maintenance, however it should not be used to represent a true overall indicator of risk for a device type.

***

Subjective terms like high, medium, low, or *sufficient, reasonable, unreasonable, substantial*, and *effectiveness* - are embedded throughout various risk writings (*words italicized* are from FDA, SUBCHAPTER H--MEDICAL DEVICES, Code of Federal Regulations, Title 21, Volume 8).

Risk assessment is generally centered on two positions: <u>subjective</u> reasoning, and measurable quantifiable <u>data</u>. These terms can represent two very different approaches to risk analysis - for example, assessing the likelihood of failure intuitively, versus a reliance on repair data. Arbitrary selection is also relied on in risk assessment.

Data, measurable and quantifiable – e.g. manufacturer, model, installation date, types and numbers of repairs, time period between repairs.

Subjective reasoning – based on an individual's experience or intuition – e.g. the relative risk of harm (low, medium, great) a device failure poses to a patient.

Arbitrary – also based on an individual's experience or intuition – often used in the context of setting parameters, e.g. determining a cost cut-off for repair analysis.

At some point in the development of risk assessment methods, decisions will necessitate making subjective and arbitrary choices.

The FDA does not set requirements for medical equipment maintenance, but does make recommendations to manufacturers regarding potential risks to patients in the design and manufacturing of equipment. It may be, however, that statements like the following have contributed to the acceptance of the likelihood of failure as a risk factor: "...the likelihood that a medical device will have problems, the likelihood of a patient experiencing harm... How frequently did the manufacturer anticipate this specific failure mode or defect would occur?" (*Factors to Consider Regarding Benefit-Risk in Medical Device Product Availability, Compliance, and Enforcement Decisions,* FDA, Center for Devices and Radiological Health, 2016).

Risk factor: Likelihood of Failure

Failure rates and types of repair (*likelihood of failure*) should be part of the evaluation of risk and contribute to determining the inclusion and frequency of scheduled maintenance. Past failures do not necessarily predict a likelihood of failure in the future. But let's assume that by using repair data, a failure rating can be arrived at for a particular device type. For example, using a quantity of 100 of a particular device type, we find a total of 25 repairs for 25 of the units during a one year period, or a 25% annual repair rate.

We might consider this 25% rate very high, and thus establish the likelihood of failure as very high. How then should we relate this to a risk assessment and maintenance strategy? If we know the consequence of failure for this device will cause serious harm to a patient, and we have established the likelihood of a failure (based on past repairs) to be highly probable, our assessment can point us to definitely including it in a maintenance program, with perhaps a short inspection interval. But what if the repair rate was 20%, 15%, 5%, or less? How then do we establish the relative likelihood of failure for a risk assessment?

But what if we have measurable and quantifiable data that can support the use of one percentage over another in assessing risk? We may be able to establish a firm device type rating if we had a large enough (How large is enough?) dataset, delineated by manufacturer, model (perhaps serial number), year installed, age, service action and parts involved. Do this, and we may better know the risk this device failure rate represents. If we can't do this, we will need to rely on subjective intuition.

The relevance of past failure data is problematic, and makes a poor risk indicator applied to an entire device type. However, this same data can be very useful in determining a service class for a specific device; the potential for critical components to fail can place a device type on a watch list for example.

Risk factor: Failure Apparent to the Operator

If the consequence of failure is high, but a failure is easily detected by the operator, is the overall risk as high as if failures are not noticeable?

Failure Apparent to the Operator, is the proposed main risk criteria alongside *Consequence of Failure* (the ability of a failure to harm a patient). Effectively, *Failure Apparent to the Operator*, says that regardless of past device failures (*Likelihood of Failure),* if a failure can be observed by the operator, the patient is at a lower risk than if a failure can go undetected.

Examples of failures more easily detected by the operator are: aneroid manometer, EKG machine, hydrocollator, standing scale.

Examples of failures not easily detected: blood warmer temperature, nurse call function, defibrillator output.

Using this risk factor forces a decision – can the operator observe failure - that moves equipment into one of two groups: devices whose failures are observable by the operator (Yes). All other

BMET and Clinical Engineer

devices - by default - are classified as having failures *not* observable by the operator (No). This reduces the risk factor of the Yes group, and raises it for the No group.

Comparing Failure Likelihood with Failure Apparent

Table 1 shows the estimated risk using a sample of 10 device types that demonstrate a range of functions, complexity, and risk. This model represents two modes of assessment, one relying on likelihood of failure, the other on a failure apparent to the operator. The table incorporates three other variables: *Consequence of Failure* (to the Patient), *Calibration and Parts Replacement*, and *Startup Self Test*. The variables indicated as having a higher level of risk are highlighted in red.

The comparison between the two columns shows very different outcomes: *Failure Apparent* generates a greater number of high risk indications than *Failure Likelihood*.

In this sample one device type shows complete agreement between both *Failure Likelihood* and *Failure Apparent* columns: the Nurse Call System.

Table 2 shows the relevant issues for each characteristic by which the devices are coded.

Critical Device	Device Name	Consequence of Failure	Cal-Adjust, Parts Replace	Failure Likelihood	Failure Apparent	Startup Self Test
		L M G	No, Yes	L M G	No, Yes	No, Yes
	Aneroid Manometer	M	N	L	Y	N
Yes	Blood Warmer	Great	Y	M	N	N
	Centrifuge	M	Y	M	Y	N
Yes	Defibrillator	Great	Y	M	N	Y
	EKG	M	N	L	Y	Y
	Hydrocollator	L	Y	M	Y	N
Yes	Nurse Call System	Great	Y	G	N	N
Yes	Patient Lift	Great	N	L	Y	N
	Standing Scale	L	N	G	Y	N
Yes	Syringe Pump	Great	Y	M	N	N

Table 1: Comparing Failure Likelihood with Failure Apparent (LMG - Low, Medium, Great)

Addendum: Journal Article Three

Critical Device	Device Name	Failure Likelihood	L M G	Failure Apparent	N, Y
	Aneroid Manometer	Case, tubing failures.	L	Visually inspect dial.	Y
YES	Blood Warmer	Calibration, cleaning.	M	Output requires test.	N
	Centrifuge	Cleaning & bearing failures.	M	Operator detect worn bearing.	Y
YES	Defibrillator	Battery, paddle failures.	M	Output requires test.	N
	EKG	Lead wires failure.	L	Recording output visible.	Y
	Hydrocollator	Cleaning, temp calibration.	M	Water gets hot.	Y
YES	Nurse Call System	Jacks, cables, buttons fail.	G	Failure not visible.	N
YES	Patient Lift	Battery & sling replacement.	L	Structure & sling visible.	N
	Standing Scale	Height bar & casters fail.	G	Failures visible to operator.	Y
YES	Syringe Pump	Cleaning issues.	M	Requires testing.	N

Table 2: Rationale for how devices are coded for two risk criteria.

Table 3 shows basic indicators for each risk criterion: *Failure Likelihood* requires several potentially subjective assessments, while *Failure Apparent* indicators offer fewer choices, based on observation.

Failure Likelihood - Indicators		Failure Apparent to operator - Indicators	
Repair rate	Is failure rate low, medium, high?	Visual indicators	
Mean time between failures	Will repairing make another failure less likely or more distant?	Audible indicators	Are there indicators that clearly show status?
Equipment durability	Does it resist breakage?	Temperature Indicators	
Components that typically fail	Are there typical component failures that could harm patient?	Output	Can operator determine if there is an output?
Critical components that might fail.	Are there components that if they failed could harm patient?		

Table 3: Comparing Failure Likelihood indicators and Failure Apparent to operator indicators.

There is no getting around the work of assessing each device type, one at a time. And there is also no way to make strictly data-based assessments that do not depend on subjective or intuitive judgements. The purpose of the risk matrix is to provide a standardized structure for visualizing the relationships of established risk characteristics – to best observe and manage the range of subjective assessments.

Using a matrix of critical characteristics, we can classify device types and determine the need for scheduled maintenance inspections. These results can then be augmented by other information such as manufacturer's maintenance recommendations, previous maintenance inspections that resulted in a repair, repair history, alerts and recall notices.

Table 4 uses the following four criteria

- Consequence of Failure - based on the device type's direct connection to life support functions.

BMET and Clinical Engineer

- Calibration Adjustments and Parts Replacement – actions required periodically, e.g. temperature adjustment, battery replacement.
- Failure Apparent to the Operator - functional indicators that are apparent to the operator, e.g. lights, output readings.
- Start-up Self Test – pass/fail test of functions on start-up.

Table 4. Every possible combination of risk factors is displayed. Sample devices are shown assessed. Any device can be assessed by selecting the appropriate level of each criteria.

Device Name	Consequence of Failure	Cal-Adjust, Parts Replace	Failure Apparent	Startup Self Test	Scheduled Maintenance
Nurse Call System Blood Warmer Syringe Pump	High	Required	No	No	Maint. Priority
Defibrillator	High	Required	No	Yes	Maint. Priority
	High	Required	Yes	No	Maint. Required
	High	Required	Yes	Yes	Maint. Required
	High	None	No	No	Maint. Required
	High	None	No	Yes	Maint. Required
Patient Lift	High	None	Yes	No	Maint. Required
	High	None	Yes	Yes	Modified Maint.
	Medium	Required	No	No	Maint. Required
	Medium	Required	No	Yes	Maint. Required
Centrifuge	Medium	Required	Yes	No	Maint. Required
	Medium	Required	Yes	Yes	Maint. Required
	Medium	None	No	No	Modified Maint.
	Medium	None	No	Yes	Modified Maint.
Aneroid Manometer	Medium	None	Yes	No	Modified Maint.
EKG	Medium	None	Yes	Yes	Modified Maint.
	Low	Required	No	No	Maint. Required
	Low	Required	No	Yes	Modified Maint.
Hydrocollator	Low	Required	Yes	No	Modified Maint.
	Low	Required	Yes	Yes	Modified Maint.
	Low	None	No	No	Modified Maint.
	Low	None	No	Yes	Maint. Not Req.
Standing Scale	Low	None	Yes	No	Maint. Not Req.
	Low	None	Yes	Yes	Maint. Not Req.

Table 4. Risk matrix.

Addendum: Journal Article Three

Defining maintenance protocol for an AEM (Alternate Equipment Management) program should include different kinds of information from many sources:

Failure rate: number per inspection interval.

Operational complexity: simple function check, or use of test equipment.

Number of periodic inspections resulting in repair.

Number of repairs not related to periodic inspections.

Identifying typical failure causes that might be addressed during a periodic maintenance inspection.

Assessing maintenance inspections that lead to a repair – thus helping to establish a need for inspections.

Manufacturer's maintenance recommendations.

Alerts and recall notices.

Unique factors can call for specific actions. The risk assessment tool is a starting point from which maintenance protocols evolve.

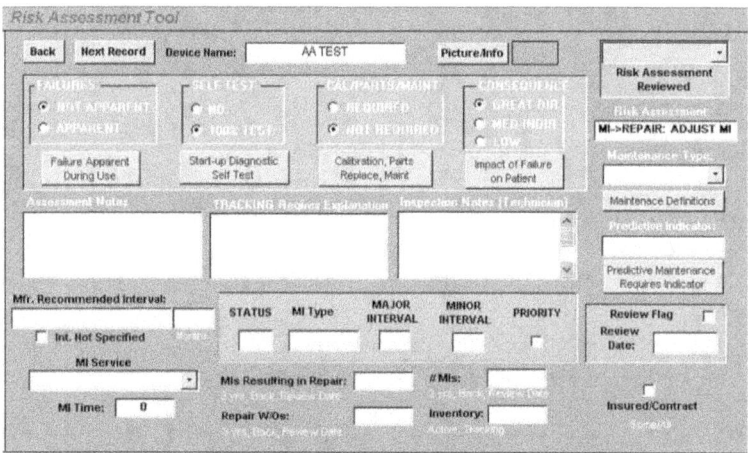

The above screenshot shows the main MS Access data input screen that was used for risk assessment at St. Luke's and Roosevelt hospitals in New York City. By selecting from the four main criteria, the database automated the risk comparisons and recommended a maintenance type and interval. That recommendation could then be altered if needed to reflect other data available to be assessed.

Below is a simplified illustration of the relationships of the various risk criteria.

BMET and Clinical Engineer

Risk	Low	Med	High
Consequence of Failure to User	LITTLE	MODERATE	GREAT
Failure Apparent to User	YES	MAYBE	NO
Cal-Adjustments Parts Replace	NO	SOME	YES
Start-up Self Test	YES	PARTIAL	NO

Other Books

Other Books by Alan Pakaln

*The Feast of San Gennaro,
Little Italy, New York, 1971*
The People, Food, Activities

B&W portraits, uncoated paper, standard printing.

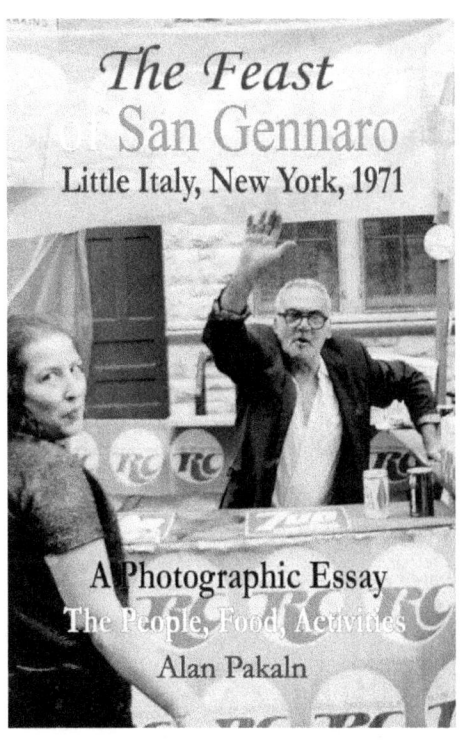

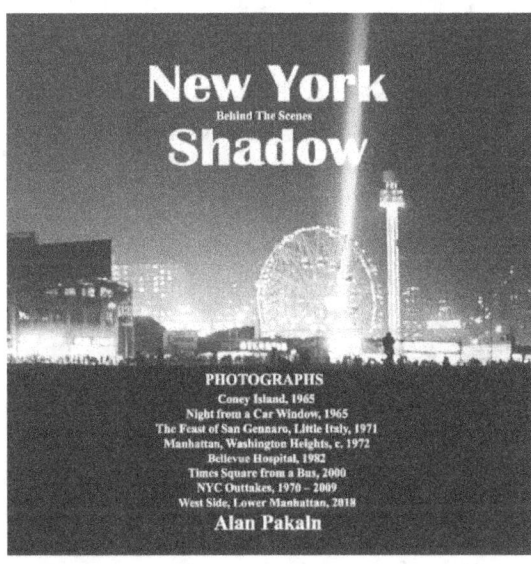

*New York Shadow:
Behind The Scenes*

Eight series
photographs
1965 through 2018
New York City
Color and B&W
Coated paper
Quality printing

BMET and Clinical Engineer

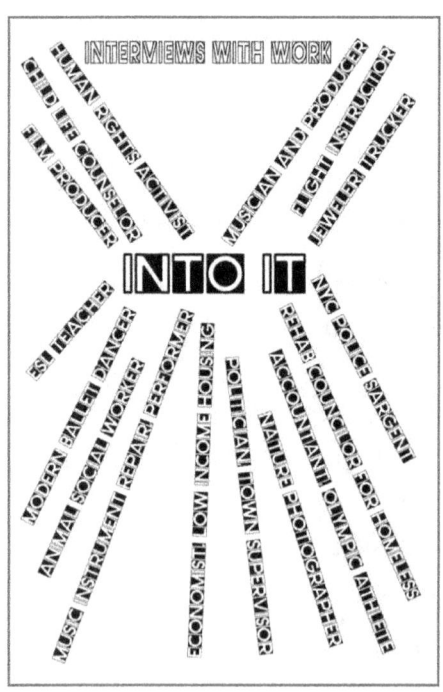

Into It:
Interviews With Work

Unusual careers worked by passionate people, e.g.: female flight instructor, Olympian accountant, South Bronx NYC police Sergeant, female jeweler truck driver.

Other Books

www.ingramcontent.com/pod-product-compliance
Lightning Source LLC
Chambersburg PA
CBHW052323220526
45472CB00001B/238